# Cutaneous Cryosurgery

Principles and Clinical Practice

Fourth Edition

# Dedication

*This book is dedicated to Dr. Rodney Dawber. Cutaneous cryosurgery owes an enormous debt to Dr. Dawber who researched, practiced, and taught the subject to a generation of young dermatologists. He inspired and co-authored the first three editions of this book which achieved an international audience. Although he is now retired from medicine, his enthusiasm for cryosurgery lives on through the pages of this book.*

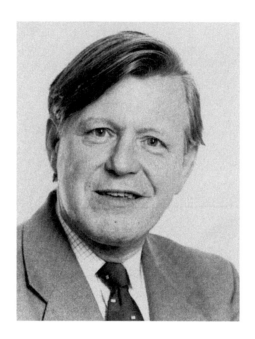

# Cutaneous Cryosurgery

Principles and Clinical Practice

Fourth Edition

**Richard P. Usatine, MD, FAAFP**
Professor, Dermatology and Cutaneous Surgery
Professor, Family and Community Medicine
Medical Director, Skin Clinic
University of Texas Health Science Center at San Antonio, Texas, USA

**Daniel L. Stulberg, MD, FAAFP**
Professor of Family and Community Medicine
Director, Preceptorship Programs, University of New Mexico School of Medicine,
New Mexico, USA

**Graham B. Colver, BM BCh, MA, DM, MRCP, FRCP(Ed)**
Dermatology, Chesterfield Royal Hospital NHS Foundation Trust, Chesterfield, UK

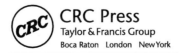

CRC Press
Taylor & Francis Group
Boca Raton London New York

CRC Press is an imprint of the
Taylor & Francis Group, an **informa** business

CRC Press
Taylor & Francis Group
6000 Broken Sound Parkway NW, Suite 300
Boca Raton, FL 33487-2742

© 2015 by Taylor & Francis Group, LLC
CRC Press is an imprint of Taylor & Francis Group, an Informa business

No claim to original U.S. Government works

Printed on acid-free paper
Version Date: 20140804

International Standard Book Number-13: 978-1-4822-1473-4 (Hardback)

**Visit the Taylor & Francis Web site at**
**http://www.taylorandfrancis.com**

**and the CRC Press Web site at**
**http://www.crcpress.com**

# Contents

# Preface

The first edition of *Cutaneous Cryosurgery* appeared in 1992 and set out to provide practical information for dermatologists and family doctors who were either already using cryosurgery or who wished to add this technique to their therapeutic options. The second and third editions were modified as new research and clinical studies became available, but also in response to comments from colleagues around the world. It has been helpful that national bodies have produced guidelines for the management of premalignant and malignant skin lesions, which include cryosurgery as appropriate treatment for some lesions; this cements the place of cryosurgery and renders *Cutaneous Cryosurgery* an invaluable practical guide.

Dr. Rodney Dawber was the chief architect of the first edition – a dermatologist who almost single-handedly brought cutaneous cryosurgery in the UK to respectability, through research and infectious enthusiasm. He had a wealth of publications to his name on all aspects of practical dermatology. It was typical of the man to be inclusive and he sought the help of Dr. Arthur Jackson, author of numerous articles on cryosurgery, who was already ahead of his time for the extensive use of cryosurgery in family medicine. In addition Dr. Graham Colver, who had trained under Dr. Dawber, was recruited as the third author. He is author of 10 books and chapters on aspects of skin cancer. Although these three physicians did not share exactly the same techniques and applications for cryosurgery, they agreed on a text for the book that represented a reasonable and safe approach to the subject. Sadly neither Dr. Dawber nor Dr. Jackson was available to be directly involved in this fourth edition. Of course some of the text and photographs from previous editions are used here so to that extent their memory lives on. It has, however, created the perfect opportunity to diversify.

For this edition, Dr. Richard Usatine was asked to be the lead author. He is a Professor of Dermatology, Cutaneous Surgery, and Family Medicine in the USA.

Although he was originally trained in family medicine, he is the Medical Director of the University Skin Clinic, as part of the University of Texas Health Science Center at San Antonio. He practices dermatology full time and works closely with his colleagues in the Division of Dermatology and Cutaneous Surgery at the University of Texas. Dr. Usatine has been the lead author of two major dermatology procedural textbooks and teaches dermatology procedures to family physicians in many settings.

Dr. Daniel Stulberg was asked to join us as the third author for this fourth edition. Dr. Stulberg has co-taught cryosurgery workshops for over 10 years with Dr. Usatine and was co-author of the last dermatology procedure book by Dr. Usatine. He is a natural fit to complete the talent and experience needed for this fourth edition. Having two new authors ensures that the emphasis, style, and content are significantly different. We have also expanded the book from seven to eleven chapters, including such new areas as the evidence behind cryosurgery and other cryosurgery methods outside of liquid nitrogen. We have adhered to the same philosophy that the contents of the entire book are agreed upon by all three authors.

The combined experience of the authors has allowed for a major change and increase in the number of clinical photographs in this edition. Research has led to a better understanding of the process of cell death and the effects at the periphery of the cryolesion, and these are discussed in the Introduction. The exponential growth in the utilization of cryosurgery, via insulated probes, for the treatment of solid tumors of the lung, kidney, and prostate has led to research to further our understanding of the complex events that occur when tissue is frozen.

This book is for use chiefly by dermatologists and family physicians but nurse practitioners, physician assistants, medical students, residents, and podiatrists will also find it useful. Appropriate management of many epidermal skin lesions, whether benign, premalignant, or malignant, should take cryosurgery into consideration. This book should also be on the shelves of plastic surgeons, head and neck surgeons, and oculoplastic surgeons among others.

Graham Colver, MD
Richard Usatine, MD
Daniel Stulberg, MD

## PERSONAL NOTE

In the mid-1990s I was working on my first skin surgery book and came across the first edition of *Cutaneous Cryosurgery, Principles and Clinical Practice*. I realized that I had come across a gem of a book providing great insight into the practice of cryosurgery based on the experiences and research of three talented men. It quickly became the major reference for the cryosurgery chapter of my first book *Skin Surgery: A Practical Guide*. Up to that point in my career, I did not realize the depth and breadth of clinical uses possible with cryosurgery. The clear text and excellent photographs in the book gave me the confidence to use cryosurgery as a therapeutic option for skin cancers. It also helped me learn the basic science behind cryosurgery, as well as how to treat benign and premalignant conditions with cryosurgery. The book explained the concept of freeze times, halo diameters, and thaw times better than any other article or book on the subject.

You can imagine my delight in 2013 when Robert Peden from Taylor & Francis publishing group contacted me to ask if I would consider being the lead author/editor of the fourth edition of this book. I learned that two of the three original authors were no longer going to be involved. My introduction to the remaining original author, Graham Colver, confirmed that he would stay on to provide the continuity and expertise needed to keep the book true to its original roots. Although I was involved in the development of two new books at the time that Robert Peden contacted me, I could not say no to this offer. At this point in my life I was already a serious medical writer and had six published medical books on the market, so why not add a third book to the two I was developing? I have never regretted saying yes to this offer.

The teaching of cryosurgery is near and dear to my heart. I have been teaching cryosurgery workshops since the year 2000 to family physicians at the American Academy of Family Physicians Scientific Assembly. My last skin surgery book called *Dermatologic and Cosmetic Procedures in Office Practice* had a robust chapter on cryosurgery. But a chapter is nothing like a whole book. We hope that you will find this book to be the gem that I found 20 years ago when looking for a resource to advance my skills of cryosurgery.

Richard Usatine, MD

# 1    Introduction: History, biology, physics, cryogens

## EARLY HISTORY

Written history does not relate the first encounters of *Homo sapiens* with cold temperatures. But in the last ice age they would have been well aware of the risks attached to prolonged exposure to extreme cold and possibly the benefits such as storage of food produce and analgesic effects. Frostbite and hypothermia have hampered exploration and warfare throughout the ages. Military campaigns have been severely prejudiced by the freezing temperatures found at high altitude and there are well-documented examples such as Hannibal's crossing of the Alps in 218 BC. To this day the destructive effects of unintentional exposure to cold are seen in climbers and polar explorers in the form of frostbite (**Figure 1.1**).

Over the last few thousand years humans have experimented with and recorded potentially beneficial outcomes of exposure to cold temperatures. The analgesic and anti-inflammatory properties were recorded by the Egyptians. A papyrus document from 3500 BC described the use of cold to reduce inflammation, particularly for fractures of the skull and trauma sustained during battle. At first glance it is not clear how ice or snow would have been available at such latitudes, but even in hot countries there were means of acquiring it. Ice could be stored, from the winter time, in ice houses where it was packed in large quantities and covered with straw or other insulating materials. Alternatively runners were sent up the mountains to acquire a fresh supply of snow or ice when it was required for medical or refreshment purposes. Ingenuity was at its foremost when methods were developed to produce ice or slush in desert areas when the extreme low temperatures at night were manipulated to freeze evaporating water. The Romans and later Iranians would dig a pit and line it with insulating straw. In it was placed a water container and the opening was covered by sun-reflecting shiny metal in the day but open to the elements at night. Evaporation at night led to ice forming around the edge of the container. This was collected and stored.

And so from very ancient times it is clear that cryotherapy, or the therapeutic use of low temperatures in medicine, was an active discipline. In the fifth century BC Hippocrates noted that cold could be used therapeutically to treat inflammation in joints and to reduce bleeding, bruising, and swelling. He also commented on the anesthetic effects of freezing. Over the next 1000 years there were attempts to move the science forward but there is scant literature on the subject. One account stands out, for it not only reiterated the known analgesic properties of cold but also emphasized the hemostatic effect. This was the wartime experience of Baron Dominique Jean Larrey, the military surgeon of Napoleon's army. During the retreat of the armies of Napoleon from Moscow in the winter campaign of 1812, he noted that a limb could be amputated almost painlessly and with minimal hemorrhage if the part concerned was covered with ice or snow before the operation took place.

## EARLY SCIENTIFIC ENDEAVOR AND CRYOGENS

Shepherd and Dawber have recorded the scientific developments in the world of subzero temperatures as applied to animal and human skin.[1] There had been little scientific advance until 1777 when John Hunter, in London, recognized the effects of low temperature applied to animal tissues, observing local necrosis, vascular stasis, and

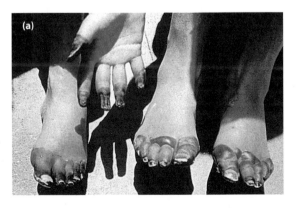
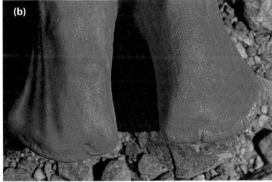

*Figure 1.1*  (a) Gangrene of digits after prolonged high altitude exposure. (b) Same digits seen 2 years later.

excellent healing. These three features of cryosurgery are equally pertinent today. Scientific observations had become more relevant after the invention of the thermometer in the early eighteenth century. It allowed researchers to strive to produce lower and lower temperatures and helped to pinpoint at what temperature certain biologic events took place. Studies on the controlled destruction of living tissue followed closely upon improved methods of generating colder temperatures. Important work on human tissue began with James Arnott, an English physician from Brighton, during the period 1845–1851. He developed a special device that allowed him to apply directly a mixture of various salts and crushed ice to achieve local temperatures of around −18°C. He demonstrated this equipment at the Great Exhibition of London in 1851 and enjoyed considerable acclaim. He used his method to treat advanced uterine tumors. This resulted in a reduction in pain, regression of the tumor, and control of symptoms. Arnott did not claim that his treatment was curative but did note some histological changes and suggested that solid carbon dioxide might be used to achieve even more effective cryotreatment. He also used cold for the treatment of cancer of the breast, headaches and neuralgia.

At the end of the nineteenth century Cailletet demonstrated the liquefaction of oxygen at the French Academy of Science and von Linde produced commercial quantities of liquid air. Dewar liquefied hydrogen in 1898 and soon developed the Dewar vacuum flask for the storage and transport of these fluids. This had the immediate benefit of allowing therapeutic use of cold liquids away from the laboratory. The first clinical application of liquid air was carried out by the dermatologist, Campbell White, in New York in 1899. The liquid was applied with a swab and used to treat skin lesions, including basal cell skin cancers, nevi, verrucae and lupus vulgaris. He was excited by the possibilities of this approach and stated: "I can truly say today that I believe that epithelioma, treated early in its existence by liquid air, will always be cured and that many inoperable cases can also be cured by its application." In 1907 Bowen and Towle reported the use of liquid air to treat pigmented hairy nevi, vascular skin lesions, and lymphangiomas. It was becoming apparent that cryotherapy of skin lesions led to better cosmetic results, with less scarring, than other treatments. Whitehouse, in 1907, developed a simple spray made from a wash bottle with two tubes through the cork and used this to treat patients with basal cell carcinomas, lupus erythematous, and vascular nevi. He treated recurrences of basal cell carcinomas after radiotherapy and found it to be more successful than repeat radiotherapy.

Around this time Dr. William Pusey, in Chicago, popularized the use of carbon dioxide snow (or carbonic acid snow) in preference to a salt and ice mixture. It had become readily available thanks to the carbonated mineral

*Table 1.1* Cryogenic Materials Used by Physicians Over the Years

| Cryogen | Introduced by | Year |
|---|---|---|
| Ice | Ancient Egyptians | |
| Ice/salt mix | Arnott | 1851 |
| Ether | Openchowski | 1883 |
| Liquid air | White | 1899 |
| Solid carbon dioxide | Pusey | 1907 |
| Freon | Hall | 1942 |
| Liquid nitrogen | Allington | 1950 |
| Nitrous oxide | Amoils | 1964 |
| Argon | Torre | 1970 |

water industry. Liquid carbon dioxide gas was supplied in steel cylinders under pressure and, when expelled into a soft material, produced a fine snow that could be molded into suitable shapes for application to the skin. One of his cases involved treating a large black hairy nevus on a young girl's face and he made the important observations that melanocytes were particularly sensitive to cold and that there was little thickening or scarring of tissues after even deep freezing techniques. He successfully treated other nevi, warts, and lupus erythematous. Pusey stated of carbon dioxide snow that "we have found a destructive application whose action can be accurately gauged and is therefore controllable." Hall-Edwards of Birmingham, in 1913, described his extensive use of carbon dioxide treatments, which was all the more remarkable because he was a respected radiotherapist. He detailed many conditions in which treatment was effective but was particularly struck by its efficacy in rodent ulcers (basal cell carcinoma.)

Carbon dioxide slush, a mixture of carbon dioxide and acetone, was used extensively for acne. As the use of carbon dioxide snow became more widespread so did the range of conditions treated. De Quervain reported the successful use of carbonic snow for bladder papillomas and bladder cancers in 1917.

Carbon dioxide cryotherapy had limitations because the lowest temperatures that it recorded on the surface were around −79°C and this did not penetrate more than 2 mm into the tissue. Nevertheless it was a great step forward and found great favor up to the 1960s. Meanwhile in the 1920s liquid oxygen became available, achieving temperatures of −183°C, and this was used by Irvine and Turnacliff to treat a range of conditions including warts, lichen planus, herpes zoster, and contact dermatitis. Its failure to achieve more widespread use lay mainly with the attendant fire risks.

Between 1920 and 1945 few advances occurred in the field. There were no technological or refrigerant advances and people concentrated on the use of carbon dioxide pencils and slush to treat conditions such as acne and post-acne scarring. Other reasons for stagnation in cryosurgery were the development of radiotherapy for cancers and the increasing sophistication of excisional surgery, together with the relative safety of general anesthesia.

### The Impact of Liquid Nitrogen

After World War II liquid nitrogen (−196°C) became widely available and Allington used this on a swab applicator to treat some benign skin lesions, including warts, keratoses, leukoplakia, hemangiomas, and keloids. Liquid nitrogen had similar properties to liquid air and oxygen but was much safer to use. Studies comparing liquid nitrogen swabs and solid carbon dioxide showed that liquid nitrogen provided more effective heat exchange, largely due to its lower boiling point. The swab method, however, has a limited freezing capacity due to its low thermal mass and the poor conductivity between swab and skin. Zacarian and Adham attempted to overcome these limitations by applying solid copper cylinders, cooled in liquid nitrogen, directly to the skin. The improved heat exchange and thermal mass enabled them to achieve freezing to a depth of 7 mm compared with the 2 mm achieved with swabs.

The next major developments in the use of cryosurgery took place in the early 1960s when various cryoprobes were developed. Cooper and Lee, in 1961, developed a liquid nitrogen (−196°C)-cooled probe that was capable of controlled freezing of tissues of the brain. The probe consisted of three concentric tubes, with the central tube carrying liquid nitrogen from a pressurized cylinder to a chamber at the probe tip where the nitrogen vaporized and gaseous nitrogen was returned via the middle channel. The outer channel consisted of vacuum insulation, which ensured that freezing took place only at the probe tip. The probe was used for neurological treatment of Parkinson's disease and other neuromuscular disorders. In 1964, Amoils and Walker developed an improved probe in which cooling was achieved by the Joule–Thomson effect on compressed nitrous oxide, for the treatment of ophthalmologic conditions. This probe provided more rapid cooling and did not require thermal insulation. Compressed gas was supplied to the probe and expanded through a small orifice, close to the probe tip. Temperatures of −70°C could be achieved and the system was highly controllable.

Douglas Torre, the New York dermatologist, developed a liquid nitrogen spray, which could be used with a variety of tips, allowing areas of different sizes to be treated. The spray could be operated with one hand and the closed system provided by the tip gave greater cooling capacity and allowed a wider range of conditions to be treated. Dr. Zacarian developed the first handheld spray in 1968. In 1968, Michael D Bryne developed the handheld "Kryospray" unit (**Figure 1.2**), which was the start of Brymill, a leading company providing cryosurgery systems

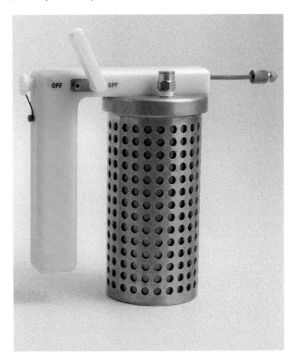

*Figure 1.2* The "Kryospray" unit was developed by Michael Bryne in 1968 as one of the first handheld cryospray units in the world. It was the start of the Brymill Cryosurgical Systems Company. (Courtesy of Craig LaPlante.)

throughout the world. This was when the term "cryosurgery" ("cold handiwork") was first used in practice. In the USA some key figures practiced and taught cryosurgical techniques once the cryospray was widely available – these included Zacarian, Torre, Gage, Kuflik, Graham, Lubritz, Elton, and Spiller. In the UK the inclusion of cryosurgery training in surgery workshops was popularized by Dawber and others, and with time the popularity of cryosurgery spread around the world. The range of lesions that can be treated with cryosurgery is now wide and includes many benign, premalignant, and malignant conditions.

## BIOLOGY OF CELLULAR INJURY

The study of cryobiology can be divided into two main areas. Cell preservation covers areas such as the preservation of blood products, gametes, embryos, and organs for transplantation. Cell destruction deals with cold-induced cell and tissue damage, and this underpins the discipline of cryosurgery. Understanding the mechanisms of cell damage is important if maximum benefit is to be gained from treatments. The tissue response to cold injury, which can range from inflammation to total destruction, depends on the severity of freezing. The lesion created by freezing is characterized by coagulation necrosis in the central region with a surrounding, relatively thin, peripheral region in which cell death is apparent. The effects are described as either early, direct or delayed, indirect. Before a detailed description is given it is important to emphasize that the effects of cryosurgery are not uniform across the treated area. In the border, or peripheral, zone the cooling rate is slow, the duration of freezing is short, the final temperature is in the range 0 to −10°C, and warming is rather rapid. In this zone, some cells are necrotic, others are apoptotic, and others may survive. Many cells close to the 0°C isotherm will survive and it is in this range that differences in cell sensitivity to freezing injury become evident. Much of the basic science in this area is "cell" science and not necessarily directly applicable to whole tissues and organs. It will be seen how delayed changes such as hypoxia then influence the damage done by the primary effects of ice formation.

### Early Effects

Cooling cells to a temperature of about −10°C causes little damage because the cell is protected for a period of time from the effects of low temperature by the cell contents, mainly the cytoplasm. As the temperature falls further, ice crystals form and this has more serious consequences for cell viability. During slower freezing, crystals initially form in the extracellular spaces at temperatures of around −15°C or below. As they form from pure water, the extracellular solute concentration increases. This creates an osmotic potential and leads to net movement of water from the intracellular to the extracellular spaces. The resulting high intracellular solute concentration damages the enzyme systems and destabilizes the cell membrane.

The second major mechanism of direct cell destruction is intracellular ice formation. This effect is more dominant with rapid cooling rates and occurs once the temperature falls to between −20 to −40°C. Rapid cooling enables ice crystals to nucleate within the cell before the process of osmotic dehydration has occurred, trapping water in the cell. The crystals damage cell organelles and membranes causing cell death. The relative importance of these two mechanisms will depend on the rate of cooling. Very rapid cooling leads to intracellular ice formation and relatively slow rates of cooling cause cell damage by solute effects. Some of these effects may be mediated by the cold denaturation of proteins, whereby the three-dimensional conformation of proteins is altered by cooling and dehydration.[2]

A further damaging effect to cell viability is found during the thawing process. Extracellular ice melts before intracellular ice, creating an osmotic fluid shift of water into damaged cells, causing swelling and bursting. Also as the temperature rises, recrystallization takes place, whereby smaller ice crystals fuse to form larger, more thermodynamically stable ones. The larger crystals have a physically damaging effect on the cell membrane. Slow or spontaneous thawing will maximize recrystallization, mechanical damage, and hence cell destruction. The temperature at which maximum intracellular ice crystal formation is found is between −20 and −25°C.[3] When the ice crystals melt, this releases a flood of pure water, causing the cell to become hypotonic for a short period and may cause the cell to burst. The damage caused by freezing will involve more than one of these mechanisms and the predominant one will depend on the time–temperature history of the tissue. In any tissue treated with cryosurgery, the temperature experienced by different areas will vary widely. Areas adjacent to a cryoprobe will attain temperatures close to the cryogen temperature, whereas areas at the periphery of the lesion will be at temperatures closer to the freezing point or normal tissue temperature. The regions will also experience different rates of cooling and warming, depending on their distance from the probe.

### Delayed Effects

The major delayed effect, which occurs some hours after cryosurgery, is vascular damage. The initial vascular response to cold is vasoconstriction followed by a cessation of blood supply as the temperature falls into the freezing range. This leads to tissue ischemia during the freezing process. As thawing takes place blood vessel endothelial cells reveal damage.[4]

This leads to platelet aggregation and microthrombus formation. The vessels become occluded, resulting in further ischemia and necrosis. The effects are greater in venules where blood flow is slower. Freezing also increases the permeability of the vessel walls and causes tissue edema. These changes enhance the hypoxic environment and lead to increased cell death.

There is evidence to suggest that some cells undergo apoptosis (gene-regulated cell death) when exposed to temperatures around −6 to −10°C. This could be an important mechanism of cell death for cells at the periphery of the ice ball, although much of the research on apoptosis and low temperatures has been carried out in vitro and its importance in vivo requires further work.[5]

### Immunological Effects

Most of the work on this topic relates to large tumors and metastases in liver, prostate, kidney, and breast cancer, but it gives insight to the mechanisms that may be important in dermatologic practice. The mechanism is thought to be the development of sensitivity to the tissue destroyed by cryosurgery. It has been proposed that larger numbers of apoptotic cells might cause tissue protection and lead to immunosuppression whereas larger numbers of necrotic cells could serve as immunostimulators.[6] More recent work has, however, shown that apoptotic cells may at times have an immunostimulatory role.[7] In another study on breast cancer and cryoablation, the rate of freezing influenced T-cell recruitment.[8] It may be that the timing of the assessment is important such that early assessment might miss antitumor activity. Later evaluation may be more relevant.[9] In dermatology, anecdotal clinical examples cited are the disappearance of distant viral warts after local freezing of a few lesions only and clearance of cutaneous metastases of malignant melanoma after freezing a solitary lesion. In the laboratory, evidence of this immunological protective effect for melanoma was found by Redondo et al.[10] They showed that cryosurgery led to destruction of implanted melanoma cells in mice and led to a 70% protection effect from attempts at further implantation. When, in addition, imiquimod was applied to the cryosurgically treated site, the degree of protection rose to 90%.

## CRYOSENSITIVITY AND MAXIMIZING CELL DEATH

In vivo experiments have shown great diversity in the sensitivity of different cell types to low temperatures with estimates of −4°C for melanocytes to −60°C for some cancer cells. However, gauging the lethal temperature for tissues as a whole is much more complex. To some extent it depends on the free water content so that skin, mucous membranes, and granulation tissue are cryosensitive whereas fibrous tissue, fat, and bone are relatively resistant. The sensitivity of melanocytes and resistance of connective tissue can be seen in freeze branding of cattle where the pigment has disappeared but there is no distortion of the treated area (**Figure 1.3**). Every facet of the freeze–thaw cycle may produce injury to the tissue, and all may be manipulated. There are five phases, and knowledge of the effect of each phase of the cycle is critical, whether the goal is complete or selective tissue destruction:

1. The rate of cooling varies throughout the tissue and only the part in direct contact with the cryogen or probe freezes at maximum rate. Slow cooling tends to produce extracellular ice, which is less destructive except perhaps in highly cellular tissues. However, some intracellular ice does form even at slow cooling rates. The cooling rate at the periphery slows as the volume of frozen tissue expands until no further expansion can occur. The cooling rate is not the most important factor.

2. The lethal temperature for a tissue is different from the cell sensitivity because secondary changes of vascular stasis and hypoxia have a major impact on survival. It is important, when dealing with neoplasms, to achieve maximum cell death and temperatures of −20°C may not be adequate.[11] Currently the consensus is that temperatures of −40°C are probably sufficient for direct killing but the secondary hypoxic changes may allow for successful cell death at the warmer, more distant parts of the tumor.

3. The practical application of the freeze–thaw cycle is discussed elsewhere but one of the measurements is the length of time that the tissue is maintained in the frozen state. Some authors pay little regard to this because they are using monitoring and aim to achieve only a certain temperature. However, experiments have shown that prolongation of the frozen state increases the destructive effect.[12] This effect may be unimportant at temperatures colder than −50°C.

4. Slow thawing enhances the destructive effect considerably and should be as slow as possible. Experience with frostbite and cryopreservation has shown that rapid warming increases the chance of cell survival.

5. If a second freezing cycle is undertaken, the ice formation upon thawing is even greater than after the first cycle, so repeat cycles are thought to be more effective at tumor destruction.[13] The interval between cycles has received little attention but if time permitted it is likely that waiting for 10 min or more would be more effective. In summary, the optimal technique for the destruction of tumors is fast freezing of the tissue to an appropriate low temperature, slow thawing, and repetition of the freeze–thaw cycle.

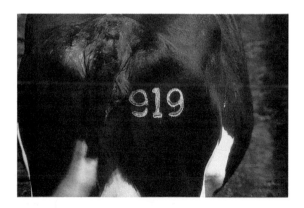

*Figure 1.3* Freeze-branded cow showing loss of pigmentation but no connective tissue distortion.

## WOUND HEALING AFTER CRYOSURGERY

The pattern of healing reflects the cryosensitivity of the tissues treated. Minor freezing injury, such as that produced by short exposure to a temperature of about −10°C, is likely to result in little tissue loss and will heal quickly. Lower temperatures are associated with degrees of tissue loss, depending on the temperature achieved and the time frame. After the production of coagulation necrosis there begins an infiltration of neutrophils, then mononuclear cells, starting at the wound edge and stimulated by the mediators of inflammation. The underlying

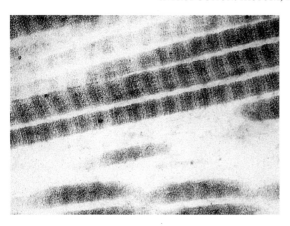

*Figure 1.4* Transmission electron micrograph of "normal-looking" collagen fibrils following cryosurgery.

collagen is relatively resistant to damage[14] as seen in the electron micrograph (**Figure 1.4**), so there remains a scaffold around which healing can take place. Granulation tissue forms, fibroblasts differentiate into myofibroblasts, and gradually normal vasculature is seen together with epithelialization.[15] Direct observation of healing using reflectance confocal microscopy has allowed researchers to visualize the process from the earliest edema and vasodilation through to the healing phase with finger-like projections into the wound bed.[16]

Clinical wound healing after cryosurgery is slow. The diseased part has been destroyed in situ and it takes time to remove all the necrotic tissue whether by slough or resorption, so healing is slow in comparison to excision and primary suture of a wound. Immediately after freezing, there is erythema and edema, often with blister formation. As necrosis sets in, the surface ulcerates and a purulent discharge occurs. This stage may last for weeks with an eschar developing, only to be shed and replaced by another as the wound gradually stabilizes. The final scar is often pale with slight atrophy but has a softer, almost normal consistency and texture. This advantageous feature of cold-induced scars is in contrast to those induced by hot thermal burns. Work on rat skin demonstrated much more collagen production in hot- compared with cold-induced burns.[17]

## PHYSICS
Research into the biology and physics of cutaneous cryosurgery has led to important areas of greater understanding but has its limitations. Experimental cryosurgery allows for control of most parameters and precise measurement. However, in vivo there are factors of infinite variability such as room and skin temperature, skin thickness, and blood flow. Tissue below the surface and at the periphery cools at a slower rate than those elements in direct contact with the refrigerant, and ice crystal formation has different effects in living tissue compared with cell suspensions.

## Shape of the Ice Ball
The shape of the expanding ice ball is important in our understanding of tissue destruction. To the novice it may appear that a visible, spreading icefield is represented, below the surface, by a similar area of ice formation. This is far from the truth. Rather than an iceberg effect, in which a greater part of the damage would be seen below the surface, there is instead a roughly hemispheric ice ball. This may not be important in the treatment of entirely superficial lesions but becomes important when treating deeper disease. The importance of this can be demonstrated by considering an infiltrative basal cell carcinoma. Its growth pattern may produce deep extensions that spread laterally beyond the visible lateral margin, whereas the depth of a therapeutic ice ball is less than the diameter of its visible lateral margin. The shape of the ice ball and the isotherms (lines linking all points of equal temperature) within it vary according to the shape and size of the probe (or spray), the rapidity of freezing, and the pressure exerted on the surface. A pointed probe, pressed lightly on the surface, produces a roughly hemispheric ice ball whereas a disc-shaped probe produces a flatter and less deep ice front. Sprays, when used with the spot freeze method, are more akin to the pointed probe initially producing a hemispheric shape. For a small increase in lateral spread there is a larger increase in depth, especially at the center. During the early stage of freezing the lateral spread of ice from the edge of the probe or cone is approximately equal to the depth of freeze (**Figure 1.5**). For this reason large lesions should generally not be treated with a single probe or spray application. It may not be possible to achieve sufficient lateral spread and, even if it were possible, it may be associated with greater deep destruction than is needed. Multiple, overlapping applications of the probe or spray are usually a better option. Another option would be a spray paint or spiral application of a cryospray (see Chapter 5).

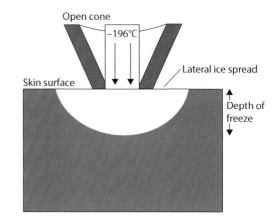

*Figure 1.5* Early on the lateral ice spread is similar to the depth of freeze.

Our knowledge of icefields comes from observation and measurement. The simplest model to observe the shape of the ice ball induced by various refrigerants is a gelatin block (**Figure 1.6**). When viewed from the side, the spreading ice ball can be seen clearly. These observations cannot be fully extrapolated to living tissues, principally because a blood supply has a profound effect on the spread of cold. Studies designed to elucidate the interrelationship of surface temperature, lateral spread, and depth of freeze have relied on thermocouple devices to monitor temperature.

When a tissue is cooled, the rate of heat exchange depends on water content, blood supply, thermal conductivity of the tissue, rate of freeze, and temperature of the refrigerant, among other variables. There are no formulae by which cell death can be predicted and further study is still required to produce ideal treatment protocols for the reproducible, consistent destruction of benign and malignant tumors. Much of the information accrued to date, which has led to the present state of the art, comes from experimental work on, for example, pigskin, with temperature monitoring and histological assessment. There are differences between the effects of a probe and a spray and between an open compared with a funneled spray technique (as with a neoprene cone). However, the important data that have led to the modern approach to cryosurgical practice can be summarized as follows:

- An open spray gives the most rapid drop in temperature. It will freeze to a greater depth than a closed probe unless pressure is exerted on the probe. However, the shape of the ice ball is approximately similar for the two methods. Up to depths of about 6 mm the contour of the ice ball is rounded but below this it becomes more triangular in shape at 1 min (**Figure 1.7**). The isotherms lie closer together when the rate of freezing is rapid.

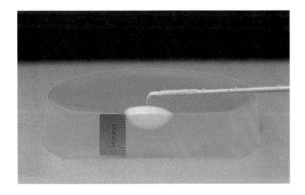

- Assessment of the actual temperature at varying depths of the skin using an open spray gives some confidence as to the killing ability of the treatment protocol. Work by Dawber and Shepherd using live pigskin with thermocouple monitoring and a surface icefield 2 cm in diameter, maintained for 30 seconds, found temperatures < −40°C at the periphery and < −50°C at least 5 mm below the surface (**Figure 1.8**).

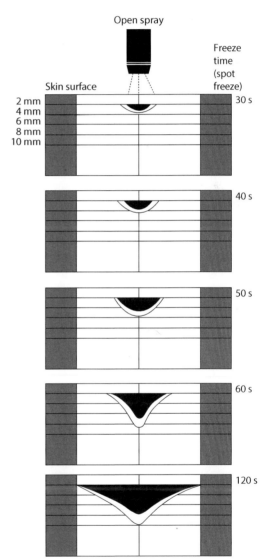

*Figure 1.6* A gelatin block (gel pad) is a simple model to observe the shape of the ice ball induced by various refrigerants. When viewed from the side, the spreading ice ball can be seen clearly. In this case, a bent tip extension has sprayed liquid nitrogen on the gel for 60 seconds, forming a hemispheric ice ball.

*Figure 1.7* Evolution of ice ball with continuous freezing. Note how the shape starts out as hemispheric and becomes more triangular with greater depth in the center at 1 min. (Adapted from Breitbart EW. Cryosurgery in the treatment of cutaneous malignant melanoma. Clin Dermatol 1990;8:96–100.)

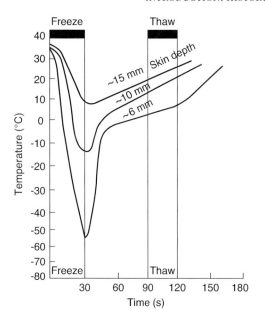

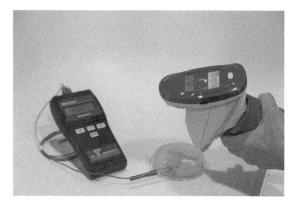

*Figure 1.9* Using thermocouple technology and infrared sensors to measure temperatures during freezing with liquid nitrogen.

*Figure 1.8* Temperatures attained at several depths below a spot freeze of 30 seconds after icefield formation using liquid nitrogen spray. Lower temperatures are obtained closer to the surface but even at 6 mm of depth the temperature does reach below −50° at 30 seconds. Note that the graph shows the temperatures during the thaw time as well.

- When dealing with malignant disease, it is important to understand the growth pattern of the tumor. Of the common basal cell carcinomas, 90% are ≤3 mm in depth; on the whole the cryosurgical techniques described in this book are recommended for such tumors. The experimental data support the concept that lethal temperatures can be readily achieved at this depth. As a result of the relationship between depth and lateral freeze, we advocate that the minimum diameter of the icefield should be about 16 mm. This diameter does of course include a margin of clinically normal skin on either side of the tumor (normally between 3 and 5 mm depending on the size and type of tumor).
- Similar general conclusions have been reached by other authorities in the field; stressing the importance of lateral spread of freeze and rapid cooling, they felt that when treating lesions 0.5–2.5 cm in diameter, a lateral spread of freeze beyond the tumor margin of 5 mm, produced within 60–90 seconds from the commencement of spraying, will give a −50°C isotherm depth of about 3 mm.

## MONITORING METHODS

The newest method to monitor cryosurgery involves the use of infrared sensing available on the Brymill Cry-Ac TrackerCam device. This is a non-invasive method of monitoring surface temperature and is discussed in Chapter 3. This method has been calibrated and tested with thermocouple technology for accuracy of measurement (**Figure 1.9**).

## CRYOSURGERY IN OTHER SPECIALTIES

Improving technology has helped to develop the dermatologic applications of cryosurgery, but in other specialties the technology has leapt forward even more. The practical applications for various anatomic sites have been reviewed by Gage et al.[18] Using ultrasound intraoperatively to monitor the accurate placement of cryoprobes, and the freezing process developed in the 1990s, allowed use of cryosurgery deep in visceral tissues. Closed cryoprobe systems have utilized multiple cryoprobes that are controlled using a computer microprocessor to allow fine-tuned control of the freezing process. Long, thin probes can be inserted deep into the prostate, lung, or kidney with percutaneous access. Commonly used cryogens are pressurized, supercooled liquid nitrogen and argon gas. Liquid nitrogen systems supercool the cryogen and then force it under pressure through the cryoprobes. In contrast, argon gas-based systems operate by supplying high-pressure gas to the cryoprobes through a Joule–Thompson port, resulting in ablative temperatures.

It is now considered useful for the destruction of hepatocellular carcinoma,[19] some renal tumors,[20] and tumors in lung, prostate, pancreas, rectum, breast, brain, and oral ·cavity.

It is interesting to read the assessment of cryosurgical practice across many disciplines by Korpan.[21] He believes that, in the future, cryosurgical techniques will be complementary to conventional surgery but also in some situations superior to it by nature of either the disease process or the condition of the patient. He reminds us that it is inexpensive and quick, and can be performed as an outpatient. However, he cautions that the apparent simplicity of the technique may lead some physicians, especially those with less experience, to deviate from the protocol and to blame poor results on the method rather than questioning their skill level or technical knowledge. This warning should be also heeded by dermatologists.

## REFERENCES

1. Shepherd J, Dawber RP. The historical and scientific basis of cryosurgery. Clin Exp Dermatol 1982;7:321–8.
2. Privalov PL. Cold denaturation of proteins. Crit Rev Biochem Mol Biol 1990;25:281–305.
3. Gage AA, Baust J. Mechanisms of tissue injury in cryosurgery. Cryobiology 1998; 37:171–86.
4. Finelli A, Rewcastle JC, Jewett MA. Cryotherapy and radiofrequency ablation: pathophysiologic basis and laboratory studies. Curr Opin Urol 2003;13:187–91.
5. Clarke DM, Robilotto AT, Rhee E, et al. Cryoablation of renal cancer: variables involved in freezing-induced cell death. Technol Cancer Res Treat 2007;6:69–79.
6. Sabel MS. Cryo-immunology: a review of the literature and proposed mechanisms for stimulatory versus suppressive immune responses. Cryobiology 2009;58:1–11.
7. Zitvogel L, Kepp O, Senovilla L, et al. Immunogenic tumor cell death for optimal anticancer therapy: the calreticulin exposure pathway. Clin Cancer Res 2010;16:3100–4.
8. Sabel MS, Su G, Griffith KA, Chang AE. Rate of freeze alters the immunologic response after cryoablation of breast cancer. Ann Surg Oncol 2010;17:1187–93.
9. Wolchok JD, Neyns B, Linette G, et al. Guidelines for the evaluation of immune therapy activity in solid tumors: immune-related response criteria. Clin Cancer Res 2009;15:7412–20.
10. Redondo P, del Olmo J, López-Diaz de Cerio A, et al. Imiquimod enhances the systemic immunity attained by local cryosurgery destruction of melanoma lesions. J Invest Dermatol 2007;127:1673–80.
11. Neel HB, Ketcham AS, Hammond WG. Requisites for successful cryogenic surgery of cancer. Arch Surg 1971;102:45–8.
12. Burge SM, Shepherd JP, Dawber RP. Effect of freezing the helix and the rim or edge of the human and pig ear. J Dermatol Surg Oncol 1984;10:816–19.
13. Whittaker DK. Degeneration and regeneration of nerves following cryosurgery. Br J Exp Pathol 1974;55:595–600.
14. Shepherd JP, Dawber RP. Wound healing and scarring after cryosurgery. Cryobiology 1984;21:157–69.
15. Gazzaniga S, Bravo A, Goldszmid SR, et al. Inflammatory changes after cryosurgery-induced necrosis in human melanoma xenografted in nude mice. J Invest Dermatol 2001;116:664–71.
16. Terhorst D, Maltusch A, Stockfleth E, et al. Reflectance confocal microscopy for the evaluation of acute epidermal wound healing. Wound Repair Regen 2011;19:671–9.
17. Li AK, Ehrlich HP, Trelstad RL, et al. Differences in healing of skin wounds caused by burn and freeze injuries. Ann Surg 1980;191:244–8.
18. Gage AA, Baust JM, Baust JG. Experimental cryosurgery investigations in vivo. Cryobiology 2009;59:229–43.
19. Callstrom MR, Charboneau JW. Technologies for ablation of hepatocellular carcinoma. Gastroenterology 2008;134:1831–5.
20. Hui GC, Tuncali K, Tatli S, Morrison PR, Silverman SG. Comparison of percutaneous and surgical approaches to renal tumor ablation: meta-analysis of effectiveness and complication rates. J Vasc Interv Radiol 2008;19:1311–20.
21. Korpan NN. A history of cryosurgery: its development and future. J Am Coll Surg 2007;204;314–24.

# 2  Use in clinical practice

## INDICATIONS

Cryosurgery is a therapeutic technique used on the skin by dermatologists, family physicians, nurses, podiatrists, and many other clinicians. All clinicians who deal with skin disease should be aware of the treatment options available and should be able to practice with a wide "surgical repertoire." Then the informed patient can be offered the most appropriate treatment. Cryosurgery is one of the options and the decision whether to use it will depend on characteristics of the lesion, patient-specific factors, and operator experience. When specific skin conditions are discussed in Chapters 8–10 it is not assumed that cryosurgery is the only option, but that it is appropriate and will achieve the desired outcome. In some cases, eg seborrheic keratosis, curettage or shave excisions may give equally good results both cosmetically and for cure rates. In other cases, there may be a specific reason to avoid more invasive techniques even if cryosurgery does not give an ideal outcome. When dealing with malignant lesions excisional surgery may produce the highest cure rates but cryosurgery still has a role for less aggressive tumors and in a palliative setting. It is paramount that the patient is aware of the benefits and risks and the comparative cure rates (where known) for different therapeutic options. Side effects may sway an individual to opt for one modality over another.

Whereas most individuals understand the concept of excisional surgery, they are less likely to readily comprehend what is intended with cryosurgery. Treatment that produces localized frostbite, leading to delayed inflammation, swelling, and necrosis, is not immediately understood by many patients. There can even be confusion about the word freezing because some people equate this with the numbing effect of local anesthetic.

### Modes of Application

Freezing refrigerants are now so portable that cryotherapy is often the easiest treatment to offer. It is literally at hand in the office and can be applied without the patient having to move.

The choice of spray, probe, or forceps may be determined by the nature of the lesion. Compressible lesions such as angiomas are best treated by a probe, so that pressure can be exerted to partially empty the vessels at the time of freezing. Forceps application is particularly suited to polypoid lesions but is also very good for anxious patients for whom the sound and feel of the spray, especially when directed to the face, causes concern. Angulated (bent) spray tips are ideal for work on the undersurface of the chin or around the canthus. The rate at which refrigerant is delivered to the skin surface can be adjusted greatly by use of various diameter spray tips.

### Epidermal Lesions

Generally, cryosurgery is best suited to the management of epidermal lesions such as keratoses. Indeed it is hard to imagine clinical practice without ready access to a liquid nitrogen source. It is a standard approach for viral warts, actinic keratosis, and molluscum contagiosum. However, keratin is a good insulator and markedly hyperkeratotic lesions will not respond so well. Bowen's disease may be amenable to treatment, but once the disease has spread down the hair shaft it is a less effective method.

### Non-epidermal Lesions

Freeze times are generally longer for lesions arising in the dermis or the appendages.

It can be very effective for acrochordons and may shrink or cure such lesions as angiomas, chondrodermatitis, labial mucoid cysts, and sebaceous hyperplasia. There are many other indications discussed in detail in later chapters. Inevitably longer freeze times will result in increased morbidity and the destructive effects of liquid nitrogen should not be underestimated.

## CONTRAINDICATIONS

### Operator Factors

Cryosurgery is a destructive treatment, which can do great harm if used inappropriately. The ease with which it can be obtained leads many to believe that it is a therapy that is simple and easy to learn. Inexperienced clinicians should be just as wary about the use of liquid nitrogen as they would be about excisional surgery. Adequate training will help to avoid the complications discussed in Chapter 11.

### Inappropriate Lesions

There are no absolute contraindications to cryosurgery but some skin lesions are better dealt with in other ways. It would be inappropriate to freeze a suspected invasive malignant melanoma because the evidence and standards of care support excisional surgery. More generally, cryosurgery should not be used without previous histologic confirmation of a diagnosis that may be malignant.

Cryosurgery should rarely if ever be used to treat morpheaform, infiltrative, micronodular, or recurrent basal cell carcinoma. Cryosurgery should not be used to treat poorly differentiated or recurrent squamous cell carcinoma.

The evidence shows poor response rates and it would only be used palliatively.

### Inappropriate Site or Skin Type

Malignant tumors in high-risk sites such as the preauricular and nasolabial areas are known to have high recurrence rates after cryosurgery. In fact the cure rates after excisional surgery are also lower, but the histology report allows the operator to go back if necessary.

Care must be taken when using longer freezing times in hair-bearing sites because permanent hair loss has been reported. Careful documentation is needed because some lesions such as seborrheic keratosis on the scalp may already have sparse hair growth and the cryosurgery may be blamed erroneously for hair loss.

The hypopigmentation, or conversely hyperpigmentation, seen after cryosurgery can be very distressing for people with Fitzpatrick skin types 4 and 5. Longer freeze times are more likely to produce these changes but, if it is possible to treat an inconspicuous test area first, disappointment can be averted.

The lower leg is renowned for poor healing especially in elderly people with poor circulation. For this reason longer freeze times may lead to tissue breakdown and very long healing times. Elderly people, especially those on steroid treatment, may have very thin skin with loss of elastic tissue. These individuals are more likely to suffer edema and bruising after cryosurgery. Distressing edema with closure of the eyes can happen after freezes of moderate length around the eyes.

### Concurrent Disease and Intolerance

There are several concurrent diseases that may adversely affect the response to cryosurgery. Cryosurgery should not be offered to anyone with a history of unexpected or unexplained reactions to this treatment modality. Other specific diseases that would greatly increase the chance of an adverse response are as follows:

- Cold-induced conditions, eg cryoglobulinemia
- Platelet deficiency
- Raynaud's disease (for acral lesions) (**Figure 2.1**)
- Collagen and autoimmune disease
- Pyoderma gangrenosum.

## ADVANTAGES OF CRYOSURGERY

### Ease of Use

There are few therapeutic interventions so easy to implement. Whether the application is by cotton swab, spray, or probe, the equipment can be at hand in the exam room for immediate use. Patients are often delighted that they do not have to book a further appointment for their procedure. There is no need for sterilization of the equipment and little in the way of wear and tear.

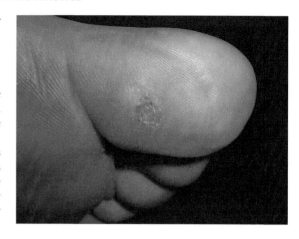

*Figure 2.1* **A plantar wart on the big toe of a patient with Raynaud's phenomenon. The physician chose to treat the patient with intralesional candida antigen rather than cryosurgery because of the patient's circulatory status. (Courtesy of Richard Usatine, MD.)**

The therapeutic effect of cryosurgery is fairly repeatable and reproducible. The techniques discussed in Chapter 5 allow treatment to be recorded and modified, as appropriate, to retreat a lesion or treat further lesions as they appear.

### Postoperative Effects

The immediate postoperative effects are usually minimal and a well-prepared patient is likely to cope with ease. After excisional surgery there are sutures to be removed, which means not only another visit but also the timing of the procedure must take into account people's travel or holiday plans. After cryosurgery, however, there will be, at most, the need for some dressings for a weeping wound. Wound infection requiring antibiotics is less common than after excisional surgery. It is unusual for patients to require time off work after cryosurgery.

Some patients have a tendency to develop hypertrophic or keloid scarring. This information is sought at the pre-assessment and may heavily sway the argument towards the use of cryosurgery. Not only is liquid nitrogen treatment very unlikely to produce this complication, but it is also part of the toolkit for managing keloids.

### Medical Conditions

There are very few circumstances in which cryosurgery, if an appropriate therapy, cannot be used. Specific contraindications are discussed earlier in this chapter. On the positive side, only slight attention has to be given to anticoagulant use, pacemakers, or patient mobility. It is suitable for those with needle phobia and individuals who cannot keep still through parkinsonism or chorea. Such individuals with involuntary movements may be at risk in excisional surgery, when sharps are a potential hazard, but equally the staff are safer especially if the patient carries a blood-borne virus.

## DISADVANTAGES OF CRYOSURGERY

### Storage and Transport

Some refrigerants can be stored over long periods of time and will always be readily available for use. Liquid nitrogen, on the other hand, evaporates and the supply must be replenished. Consequently liquid nitrogen, the most versatile cryogen, may not be cost-effective for some office clinicians who rarely use cryosurgery. In addition there are health and safety protocols to be followed for the transport of the liquid nitrogen. A clinician should not carry a loaded cryospray in his or her car. This means that a clinician who works from two offices would need to have the full storage equipment installed at both sites, with additional costs being incurred.

### Is Histology Required?

Cryosurgery is a destructive technique and provides no specimen for histologic examination. It is inappropriate to blindly treat a possible malignancy in this way. If the diagnosis is not known, it is best not to treat blindly even for benign-looking lesions.

### Postoperative Effects

The postoperative effects and complications of cryosurgery are discussed in Chapter 11 but it is important to note that the extent to which these should be regarded as a disadvantage of treatment will depend on other variables, eg hypopigmentation may be less of an issue to a fair-skinned individual but of great import to someone with dark skin. Some individuals would be worried by the possibility of prolonged post-cryosurgical edema of the eyelid, for example, and would opt for curettage or excision of a lesion instead.

Cryosurgery may cause significant pain both at the time of application and for some minutes afterwards. There is marked interpersonal variation but some sites such as the scalp and nose may be especially painful. In addition some individuals are quite anxious about a noisy, painful spray being applied to areas around the eyes, nose, and mouth. Fortunately, there are options such as topical or local anesthesia to prevent the pain of cryosurgery (see Chapter 5 for details). Also, there are cryoprobes that are an alternative to cryospray (see Chapters 3–5 for further information). An informed clinician can present the best options for treatment to the patient and an informed patient can then make intelligent decisions about the best technique for cryosurgery when cryosurgery is the treatment of choice.

# 3 Liquid nitrogen equipment

Liquid nitrogen is the preferred cryogen for performing cryosurgery of the skin. In order to work with liquid nitrogen in the office, a holding container and dispensing device are necessary. Although liquid nitrogen can be dispensed into a cup and applied with a cotton-tip applicator, this is not sufficient for the full range of cryosurgery demonstrated in this book. Therefore it is crucial to purchase a portable cryospray unit with appropriate tips and probes. It is also important to find a reliable company to deliver the liquid nitrogen to the office on a regular basis. Box 3.1 lists the main equipment necessary.

*Table 3.1* MVE Lab Series

| Size (L) | Model | Static holding time (weeks) | Weight empty (lb) | Weight full (lb) |
|---|---|---|---|---|
| 5 | 501-5 | 4–5 | 8 | 17 |
| 10 | 501-10 | 6–8 | 13 | 30 |
| 20 | 501-20 | 8–12 | 19 | 53 |
| Long Last 20 | 501-20SC | 220 days | 19 | 53 |
| 30 | 501-30 | 14–16 | 26 | 77 |
| 50 | 501-50 | 14–17 | 34 | 123 |

Static holding time refers to the amount of time liquid nitrogen will remain in the Dewar if no liquid nitrogen is withdrawn.

---

*Box 3.1* Main Equipment for Liquid Nitrogen

- Dewar (holding container)
- Dispensing device
- Cryogun (spray gun)
- Cryo Tweezers (for skin tags)
- Various tips and probes

---

## DEWARS

The holding containers come in various sizes from 5 liters to 50 liters (**Figure 3.1**). Table 3.1 gives information on various Dewar containers in the MVE Lab series, which are superinsulated for long holding times. Choose one that will be sufficient for your practice. In our practice we have the long-lasting 20 L Dewar that we keep on wheels for easy mobility (**Figure 3.2**).

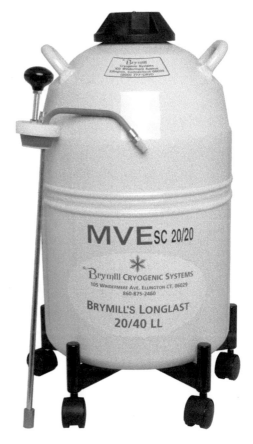

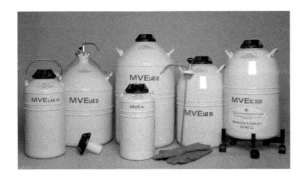

*Figure 3.1* Dewars for storage of liquid nitrogen in the office come in sizes from 5 L to 50 L. (Courtesy of Brymill.)

*Figure 3.2* A 20 L Dewar on wheels with a dispensing tube. (Courtesy of Brymill.)

## DISPENSING DEVICES

There are three major types of dispensing device:

1. A simple dispensing tube device that is held in a Dewar with some pressure applied (**Figure 3.3a**). The pressure of the evaporating liquid nitrogen in the Dewar pushes the liquid nitrogen up the tube and into the cryogun using the simple laws of physics. Although this can be done safely without protective gloves, official recommendations include wearing gloves while dispensing the liquid nitrogen. This is our preferred dispensing device because its use results in less loss of liquid nitrogen and it is less likely to break. There are no moving parts, valves, or gauges (**Figure 3.4**).

2. A spout has a pressure valve attached to the top of the Dewar and is opened for liquid nitrogen delivery (**Figure 3.3b**). Although this may appear to be the best method of dispensing liquid nitrogen, there is greater loss of liquid nitrogen from a Dewar with this set-up than with intermittent use of the long dispensing tube. These pressure valve devices are prone to breaking and can be costly to fix or replace.

3. A small long-handled ladle to scoop liquid nitrogen out of the Dewar. This is very inconvenient for anything but small amounts of liquid nitrogen to be placed in a cup. There is a significant risk of spilling due to the long handle and gloves are recommended for this process.

### Cryoguns

A cryogun is the critical equipment needed for performing cryosurgery. The major manufacturers are Brymill, Premier, and Wallach. Brymill has the widest range of cryospray tips and cryoprobes, but all cryoguns are capable of delivering liquid nitrogen by spray method to the

**(a)**

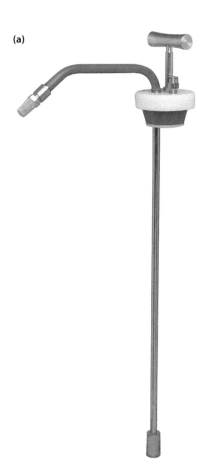

**(b)**

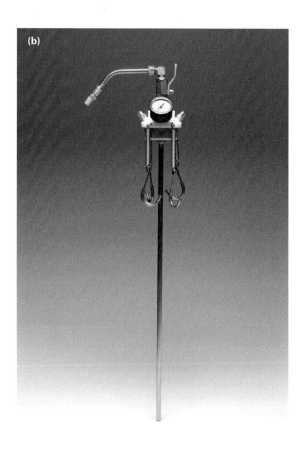

*Figure 3.3* (a) Simple dispensing tube for easy and safe dispensing of liquid nitrogen from a Dewar. (b) Dispensing device with on and off handle and a pressure gauge. (Courtesy of Brymill.)

skin. The newest cryogun by Brymill has the capability of tracking skin temperature and time while recording the procedure on high-definition video.

The Premier Nitrospray has a Luer lock connector for easy insertion or changing of the various probes and spray tips (**Figure 3.5**). Wallach makes the "UltraFreeze Liquid Nitrogen Sprayer," which comes in 500 mL and 300 mL sizes (**Figure 3.6**).

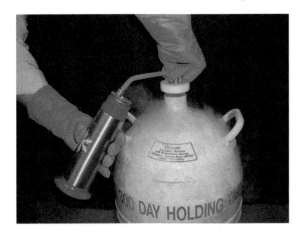

*Figure 3.4* Dispensing tube being used to dispense liquid nitrogen into a cryospray unit. (Courtesy of Richard Usatine, MD.)

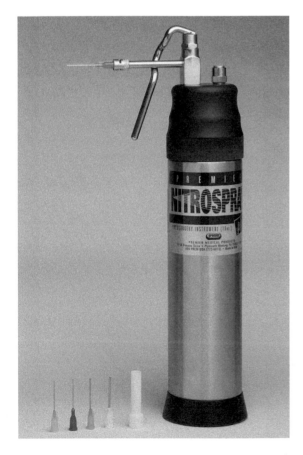

*Figure 3.5* Premier Nitrospray Plus device with Luer Lock tip. (Courtesy of Premier.)

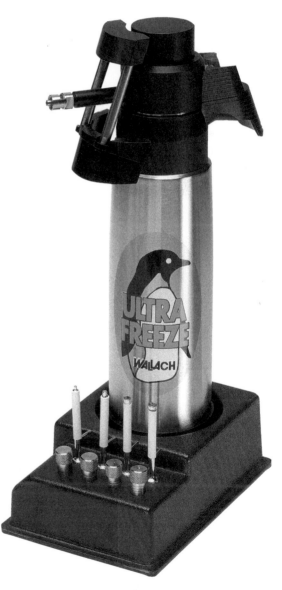

*Figure 3.6* Wallach UltraFreeze Liquid Nitrogen Sprayer with various tips. (Courtesy of Wallach.)

Michael D Bryne developed one of the first handheld spray devices using liquid nitrogen for medical use in 1968. His family continues to run the Brymill Corporation that sells the most widely used cryoguns. The variety of cryoguns available from Brymill includes (**Figure 3.7**):

- Cry-Ac: standard 500 mL capacity – the main work-horse unit.
- Cry-Ac-3: smaller capacity of 300 mL – easy handling with shorter holding time.
- Cry-Ac TrackerCam: a new device that measures the temperature of the skin when spraying liquid nitrogen using infrared sensor technology (**Figure 3.8**). See below for more detailed information.

**Spray Tips**

The original cryospray tips by Brymill came in four aperture sizes ranging from A to D. The addition of bent spray tips allows for greater versatility in cryosurgery. These tips attenuate the flow of liquid nitrogen and therefore produce a more gentle spray, which is easier to tolerate for children and sensitive adults. Also the directionality provided by the bent tip allows for spraying liquid nitrogen in any direction while keeping the spray gun vertical (tilting the spray gun may result in loss of liquid nitrogen through the top vent, which can be shocking to the patient

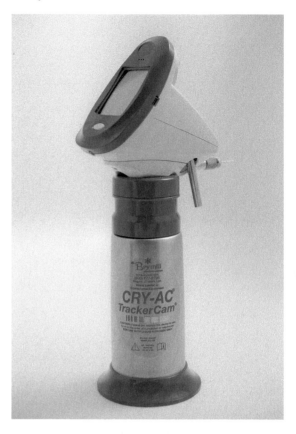

*Figure 3.8* Cry-Ac TrackerCam measures the temperature of the skin using infrared sensor technology while performing cryosurgery. (Courtesy of Brymill.)

and clinician because it often comes as a surprise with significant spray and noise).

The tips that are available for the Brymill cryoguns include:

- Four spray tips with round apertures from 0.04 inches to 0.016 inches: A is largest and D is smallest (**Figure 3.9**). The C tip has always been a favorite aperture diameter for dermatologic cryosurgery because the liquid nitrogen flow is often optimal with this tip.
- Long 20-gauge bent spray with blue cover: the longer tube (3 inches) with a 90° angle attenuates the flow of the liquid nitrogen so that the spray is less shocking to the patient (Figure 3.9). This is good for children and adults who are afraid of this therapy. It also allows for pinpoint accuracy on smaller lesions and can be rotated 360° for greater precision when treating hard-to-reach lesions. It helps to use this tip on sensitive areas such as the lips (**Figure 3.10**).

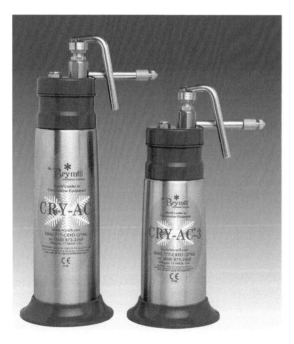

*Figure 3.7* Brymill Cry-Ac and Cry-Ac-3 cryoguns. (Courtesy of Brymill.)

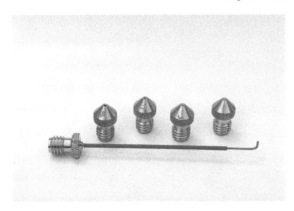

*Figure 3.9* Spray tips with apertures A–D and one bent spray tip. (Courtesy of Brymill.)

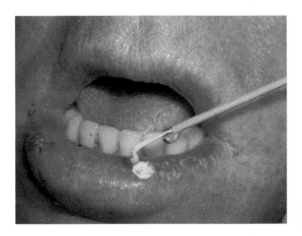

*Figure 3.10* Using a bent spray tip to treat actinic cheilitis. The 90° angle helps to deliver the liquid nitrogen efficiently to the lower lip. The bent spray attenuates the flow making this less painful than a straight tip. (Courtesy of Richard Usatine, MD.)

- Straight spray extensions (1.5–3 inches) with 16 g, 18 g, and 20 g diameters (**Figure 3.11**). These can be used anywhere on the skin or for lesions in body orifices. Straight spray-type tips allow for precise delivery of liquid nitrogen at various lengths from the cryogun. The shorter ones can be used for all kinds of lesions and the longer one can be helpful when freezing genital and perianal condylomas. It can be helpful for anogenital condylomas because it allows the clinician to be further from the lesions being treated (**Figure 3.12**).
- The "Advanced Acne Aperture" gives a soft, vaporized spray for superficial desquamation of the

cheeks, forehead, and back area in the treatment of acne. We personally do not use this method of treating acne but the spray tip is made for optimal liquid nitrogen delivery to a larger surface area.

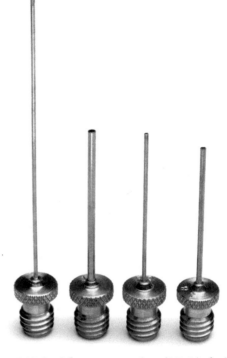

*Figure 3.11* Straight spray extensions (1.5–3 inches) with 16 g, 18 g, and 20 g diameters. (Courtesy of Brymill.)

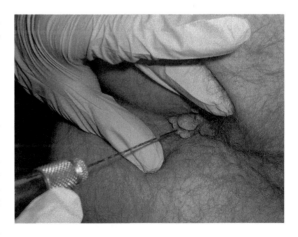

*Figure 3.12* Three-inch straight spray extension being used to treat perianal condyloma accuminata. (Courtesy of Richard Usatine, MD.)

## Cryoprobes for Liquid Nitrogen

Cryoprobes come in all shapes and sizes (**Figure 3.13**). They can easily be recognized by the clear tubes, which are needed to vent the liquid nitrogen away from the treatment area. Most of the probes are round in shape but some are conical, rounded, angled, or pointed.

These probes are helpful when treating vascular or cystic structures that respond better to cryosurgery when they are simultaneously compressed and frozen. Examples of these lesions include angiomas, mucoceles, and venous lakes (**Figure 3.14**). As this may be considered a more advanced form of cryosurgery, these tips may not

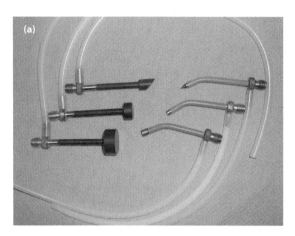

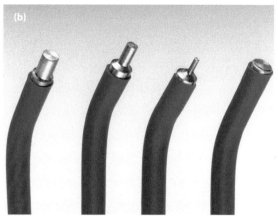

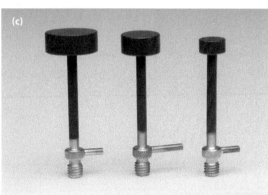

*Figure 3.13* (a) Closed cryoprobes with different shapes and sizes to apply simultaneous pressure and freezing. These are especially helpful when treating vascular lesions. The liquid nitrogen is vented out by the white plastic tube. (Courtesy of Richard Usatine, MD.) (b) Small cryoprobes. (Courtesy of Brymill.) (c) Larger cryoprobes. (Courtesy of Brymill.)

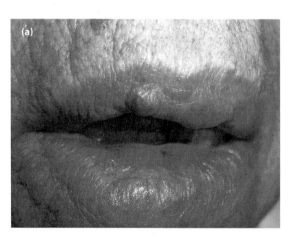

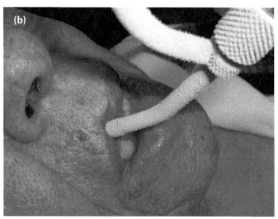

*Figure 3.14* (a) Venous lake before cryosurgery. (b) Cryosurgery of venous lake using cryoprobe to apply simultaneous pressure with freezing. (Courtesy of Richard Usatine, MD.)

be needed in the initial purchase of equipment for liquid nitrogen cryosurgery.

### Cryo Tweezers

Cryo Tweezers are designed to freeze skin tags without the overspray and inaccuracy inherent in spraying these small raised lesions. Cryo Tweezers have a Teflon-coated brass tweezer end that holds the cold temperature after dipping them in liquid nitrogen (**Figure 3.15**). They have a thin "necked" portion between the heavy tweezer ends and the handle to minimize the cold spread up the handle. The tweezers should be dipped into a Styrofoam cup with liquid nitrogen so that the tips are covered, but not the handles. The initial dip should be long enough that the liquid nitrogen has stopped boiling away from the originally warm tweezer tips (about 20 s). The handle will still get cold so some providers wrap them in a 4 × 4 gauze as they are pulled out of the liquid nitrogen. Alternatively, a thick insulated glove can be used to handle the Cryo Tweezers. The need for additional insulation can be minimized by submerging just the head of the tweezers. The skin tags are then grasped and held with the Cryo Tweezers until the freeze margin reaches normal tissue at the skin surface. The tweezers can be used to treat many more skin tags before they warm up. Re-dip the tweezers when you note that the freeze time is lengthening for additional lesions.

Cryo Tweezers are particularly good for skin tags or warts on the eyelids. After grasping the elevated papule, pull the whole lid away from the eye to protect the globe from cryodamage (**Figure 3.16**). Then continue the freeze until the whole tag or wart is white to the base. This avoids any spray possibly entering the eye. Cryo Tweezers can be cleaned between patients by allowing them to reach room temperature, and wiping with an alcohol wipe. Some clinicians use standard surgical forceps or heavy hemostats, but these do not retain the cold as long and require frequent re-dipping in the liquid nitrogen.

### Cryoplate and Neoprene Cones

Although we believe that cryosurgery is best performed by learning to control the spray using appropriate tips and techniques, many clinicians prefer to control the treatment with spray-limiting devices such as the cryoplate, ear specula, and neoprene cones (**Figures 3.17 and 3.18**). The drawback to these devices is that they limit the treatment to various geometries even though lesions come in all shapes and sizes.

The Cryoplate is a transparent plate with four conical openings of various diameters (3, 5, 8, and 10 mm) (Figure 3.17). Any spray tip can be used to spray liquid nitrogen into one of these openings for warts and other lesions (**Figure 3.19**). Cryocones come as a set of six neoprene cones of various sizes used to concentrate spray within a limited area (Figure 3.18). They can be used for irregularly shaped lesions because they can be shaped to the lesion. Sizes are 6, 11, 16, 25, 30, and 38 mm.

Learning to use the cryospray like a paintbrush is a valuable skill. Also, when the spray is spreading further beyond the lesion than desired, the cryospray gun trigger can be used in a pulsatile manner to control the halo diameter. This use of a paintbrush technique and intermittent spray obviates the need for a limiting device.

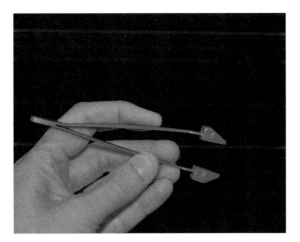

*Figure 3.15* Cryo Tweezers at room temperature. (Courtesy of Richard Usatine, MD.)

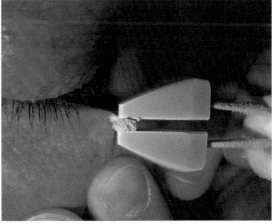

*Figure 3.16* Cryo Tweezers treating a filiform wart on the lower eyelid. Note how the wart has turned white. The Cryo Tweezers are holding the wart away from the eye with gentle pressure. (Courtesy of Richard Usatine, MD.)

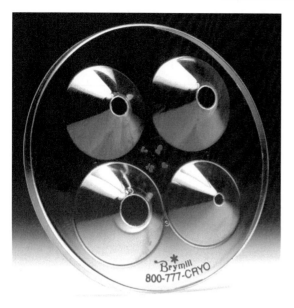

*Figure 3.17* Cryoplate with four different size apertures for controlled freezing diameters (3, 5, 8, and 10 mm) (Courtesy of Brymill.)

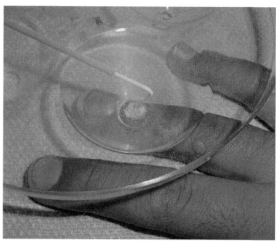

*Figure 3.19* Cryoplate being used to treat warts on the hand of a 9-year-old boy. A bent tipped spray can be helpful in this treatment. (Courtesy of Richard Usatine, MD.)

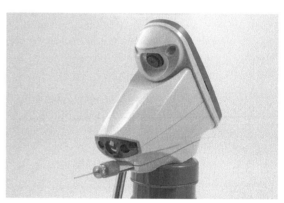

*Figure 3.20* Cry-Ac TrackerCam showing the infrared sensor, lights, and video camera. (Courtesy of Brymill.)

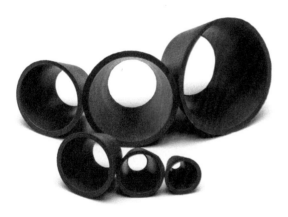

*Figure 3.18* Cryocones come as a set of six neoprene cones of various sizes used to concentrate spray within a limited area. These can be used for irregularly shaped lesions because they can be shaped to the lesion. Sizes are 6, 11, 16, 25, 30, and 38 mm. (Courtesy of Brymill.)

### Cry-Ac TrackerCam (Figures 3.20–3.22)

The Cry-Ac TrackerCam is a cryospray device that measures the temperature of the skin using infrared sensing technology when spraying liquid nitrogen on the skin. The unit is capable of recording the full treatment process in high definition video. The video is recorded on a 2-GB Mini SD memory card. To view a recording, the Mini SD Card must be removed and connected to a computer.

The right focal distance is obtained when the two blue light beams are brought together on the lesion to be treated (**Figure 3.23**). The spray is started and the upper section of the screen and the two blue beams change to GREEN when the temperature of the ice ball reaches 0°C. The upper section of the screen and the two green beams change to RED when the temperature of the ice ball reaches $T_{min}$. The temperature number is also visible in the top left corner of the screen during the procedure. The temperatures are recorded on the video so they can be seen when playing back the video on the computer. Although there are limited data to know the optimal freeze temperatures, Brymill provides temperature guidelines with the device (Table 3.2).

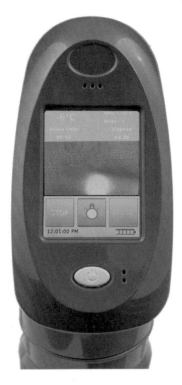

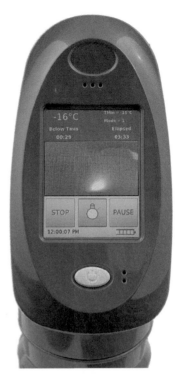

*Figure 3.21* Cry-Ac TrackerCam screen during a freeze of −6°C. Note that the green color on the screen is present at skin temperatures of less than 0°C. (Courtesy of Brymill.)

*Figure 3.22* Cry-Ac TrackerCam screen during a freeze of −16°C. Note that the red color on the screen is present at skin temperatures of less than $T_{min}$ currently set at −10°C. (Courtesy of Brymill.)

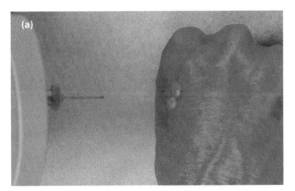

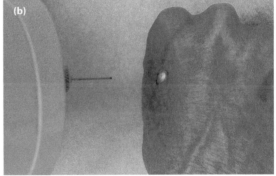

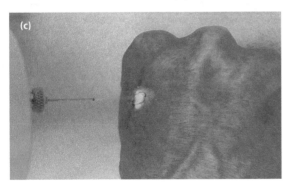

*Figure 3.23* Cry-Ac TrackerCam: (a) focusing of blue lights; (b) distance is correct when the two blue lights converge into one; (c) the light has turned green now that the skin temperature is below 0°C. (Courtesy of Daniel Stulberg, MD.)

*Table 3.2* Brymill Recommended $T_{min}$ Settings for Various Skin Lesions Using Cry-Ac TrackerCam

| Type of lesion | $T_{min}$ setting (°C) | Freeze time (s) |
|---|---|---|
| Actinic keratosis | −5 | 5 |
| Common warts | −10 | 10 |
| Cutaneous horn | −10 | 10–15 |
| Dermatofibroma | −15 | 20–30 |
| Hypertrophic scar | −20 | 20 |
| Keloid | −30 | 20–30 |
| Myxoid cyst | −20 | 20 |
| Pyogenic granuloma | −10 | 15 |
| Skin tags | −5 | 5 |
| Solar lentigo | −5 | 5 |

It is helpful to have the Cry-Ac TrackerCam to develop confidence in the treatment of appropriate skin cancers with cryosurgery. Based on expert opinion and previous thermocouple data, it appears that skin cancers should be treated to temperatures below −40°C.[1] The 30-second freeze times recommended in Chapter 10 are total freeze times and not the amount of freeze time at a temperature below −40°C. To reach a cold temperature faster it helps to use a B or C tip aperture or a straight needle tip (1 inch × 20 gauge). Do not use a bent spray tip for treating skin cancer because the flow rate of liquid nitrogen is slower and the Cry-Ac TrackerCam does not work with the geometrical configuration of a bent tip spray.

## CONCLUSION

Liquid nitrogen is the most versatile cryogen for cryosurgery. Start with the basic equipment and build over time as your cryosurgery skills advance.

## REFERENCE

1. Gage AA, Baust JM, Baust JG. Experimental cryosurgery investigations in vivo. Cryobiology 2009;59:229–43.

# 4  Equipment for other agents

In addition to the use of liquid nitrogen for cryosurgery, there are a number of different systems to achieve the low temperatures necessary for tissue destruction. The different systems each have their positive attributes as well as their limitations. Some of these tools are very portable and some are relatively inexpensive to initiate into a practice. Based on the nature of a practice and its location and access to supplies, there can be distinct advantages to the different types of equipment (Table 4.1).

## COMPRESSED GAS SYSTEMS

Releasing a compressed gas will cause a decrease in temperature. There are two types of devices that take advantage of this property. In devices that have been available for decades, the decrease in temperature can be transmitted to an adherent metal probe, which is used to perform cryosurgery. More recently some highly portable units have been developed that directly spray the gas onto the lesion, freezing the tissue.

## COMPRESSED GAS-ADHERENT METAL PROBE UNITS

There are a number of manufacturers that produce cryoguns that will attach to a gas cylinder to use in cryosurgery (**Figure 4.1**). Nitrous oxide is used more commonly than

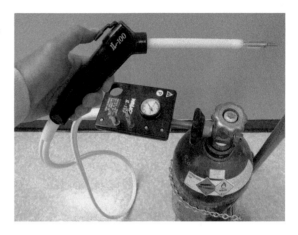

*Figure 4.1* **Nitrous oxide cryogun (Courtesy of Daniel Stulberg, MD.)**

carbon dioxide because it achieves colder temperatures more quickly, and hence treatment is faster. The nitrous oxide and carbon dioxide tanks can be refilled from a medical gas supplier or some providers have obtained the gas from other commercial sources including welding supply companies.

*Table 4. 1* Advantages and Disadvantages to Cryosurgery Devices

| Device | Time efficiency | Portability outside of primary location | Initial cost | Ongoing cost | Status of cryogen between uses | Ease of use in practice | Storage considerations |
|---|---|---|---|---|---|---|---|
| Liquid nitrogen | Excellent | Fair[a] | Moderate | Low | Evaporates | Excellent | Needs ventilation |
| Compressed gas cryoguns | Very good | Poor | Moderate | Low | No loss | Good | Bulky and heavy |
| Cryoprobe | Very good | Excellent | Moderate | Low | Gradual loss once activated | Good | Compact |
| Cryomega | Very good | Excellent | Low | Moderate | Gradual loss once activated | Very good | Compact |
| Refrigerant liquids | Fair | Excellent | Low | Moderate | No loss | Good | Compact |
| Electrical refrigeration | Very good | Fair | High | Low | No loss | Good | Tabletop, needs electricity to reach temperature |

[a]Consult local rules and regulations regarding transport of small quantities of liquid nitrogen.

The advantages to compressed gas systems using adherent cryoprobes are as follows:

- One can get excellent control of cryotherapy using different shaped tips.
- There is no concern for overspray when performing cryotherapy near sensitive structures.
- Multiple lesions can be treated relatively quickly.
- Some of the devices have a short shaft, which is easier to control for freezing skin lesions (**Figure 4.2a**).
- There is also a longer shaft (**Figure 4.2b**) available, which is useful when using the device for cryosurgery of the cervix for cervical dysplasia, or through an anoscope for cryosurgery of hemorrhoids.
- The initial cost is moderate for the equipment, the per lesion cost of supplies is very low, and the cryogun is very durable if it is not misused.
- If the provider closes off the valve of the compressed gas cylinder, the gas supply will last indefinitely. This could be useful if the provider is working in a remote area without easy access to supplies.
- Having an extra tank is useful so that, if the first tank runs out, the second tank can be installed without losing any clinical procedure time waiting for a refill. The second tank cost is low and it should be stored in a safe location in an upright position.

The following are the disadvantages to these systems:

- The tanks are large and heavy and the upfront cost is moderate.
- The probes come in a finite collection of shapes and sizes and lesions come in an infinite number of shapes and sizes.

- These units are not as fast as, and do not achieve as low a temperature as, liquid nitrogen.
- A nitrous oxide device will reach −95°C. The carbon dioxide unit will reach −70°C. Both of these are adequate for routine cryosurgery but should not be used on skin cancers because they do not achieve a cold enough temperature.
- Nitrous oxide is an anesthetic gas and a small study showed an association of nitrous oxide with miscarriage, so it should be used in a well-ventilated area, especially if for prolonged use.[1]

## COMPRESSED GAS DIRECT SPRAY UNITS

Nitrous oxide can be obtained in small metal cartridges approximately 3–4 inches in length. These disposable cartridges can be inserted into a reusable holder for cryosurgery (**Figure 4.3**). More recently a disposable plastic device has become available containing one of the nitrous oxide cartridges and the entire device is disposed of when the cartridge is empty (**Figure 4.4**).

The advantages to the direct spray units are that they are handheld, weighing less than a pound (half a kilogram), and are extremely portable. These devices travel well if the provider is based at multiple clinics. The reusable device is moderately expensive upfront but the replacement cartridges are very inexpensive. The disposable device will treat a moderate number of lesions based on the size and depth of the lesions. The upfront cost is less, but the ongoing cost of usage is higher.

The disadvantage to both of these units is that they are not quite as fast as liquid nitrogen. The temperature at −95°C is not as cold as liquid nitrogen and should not be used for skin cancers. The units sometimes develop a trail of frost between the tip and the lesion during usage. Moving the spray around can reduce this somewhat.

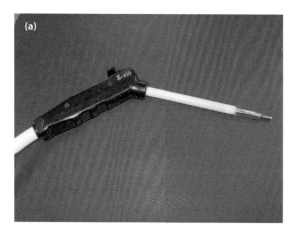
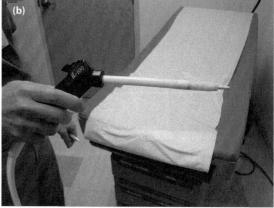

*Figure 4.2* (a) **Nitrous oxide cryogun with short shaft. (b) Nitrous oxide cryogun with long shaft for cryosurgery that is useful for cervical treatment. (Courtesy of Daniel Stulberg, MD.)**

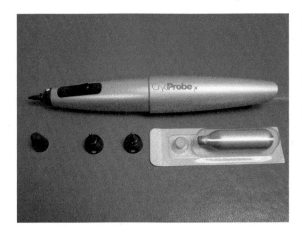

*Figure 4.3* Cryoprobe nitrous oxide spray with multiple sizes of tips. (Courtesy of Daniel Stulberg, MD.)

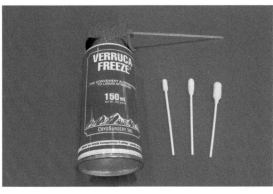

*Figure 4.5* Verruca Freeze is an evaporative liquid spray cryogen that has a hollow plastic tube for delivery or may be used with foam buds. (Courtesy of Daniel Stulberg, MD.)

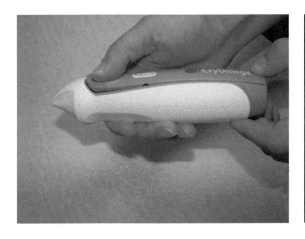

*Figure 4.4* Cryomega nitrous oxide spray unit that is disposable. (Courtesy of Daniel Stulberg, MD.)

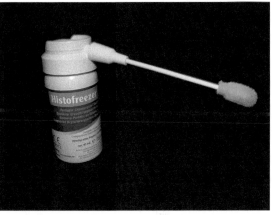

*Figure 4.6* Histofreezer with spray through swab for refrigerant liquid cryosurgery; note frost build-up on swab. (Courtesy of Daniel Stulberg, MD.)

## REFRIGERANT LIQUIDS

When liquids evaporate they induce cold temperatures. Several manufacturers produce aerosol-type canisters containing rapidly evaporating liquids (dimethyl ether, propane, and isobutene, for example) (**Figures 4.5 and 4.6**). These can be used in two ways to perform cryosurgery. In one technique the liquid is sprayed into a restricting cone and allowed to evaporate off, causing a very localized and effective freeze. The other option is to use the refrigerant liquid to cool a swab and then touch the swab to the lesion to affect cryosurgery. Several over-the-counter (OTC) versions are now available for home use (**Figure 4.7**). These OTC devices cool a foam device that can be used like a swab to freeze warts. Efficacy of these devices is difficult to know based on home use. No published studies for efficacy were found on literature review, but searching Amazon.com for "Compound W Freeze Off

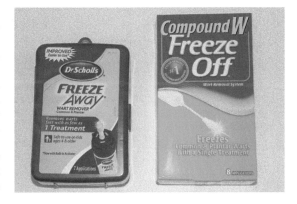

*Figure 4.7* Over-the-counter cryosurgery units. (Courtesy of Daniel Stulberg, MD.)

Wart Remover" customer reviews showed 20 people who successfully treated their warts (including 1 person with facial warts and 1 with genital warts, which are not recommended for the OTC product), 3 with success with some of their warts, 12 unsuccessful, 8 with success but commented that they exceeded the recommended treatment time or frequency, and 2 who successfully treated skin tags which is off-label. Three OTC devices were tested and reached temperatures of −20 to −23°C in contrast to beyond −100°C for liquid nitrogen.[2]

Advantages to these devices are that they are very portable and have a very inexpensive upfront cost. Once the canister is empty it is disposed of, so the ongoing cost is more expensive than for some of the other products. The control of the application of cryogen with these devices is not as tight as the adherent probes. Treatment of multiple lesions is not quite as fast with this equipment as with liquid nitrogen spray. It is similar in speed to the compressed nitrous oxide-adherent probes. These units reach −72 to −90°C, but tissue temperatures are not as low so they should not be used for cryosurgery of cancers. The size and shape of the treatment area are constrained by the size and shape of the restricting cones (when the liquid evaporation method is used).

## ELECTRICAL REFRIGERATION

This desktop unit plugs into a routine electrical outlet and uses linear compression technology to refrigerate a metal core down to −95 to −105°C (**Figure 4.8**). The metal core is then inserted into a plastic holder with an attached metal tip. There are several tip sizes available to treat various sized lesions.

Advantages to this unit are that there are no significant supplies to restock or dispose of, so it does not require delivery of liquid nitrogen on a regular basis or new gas cylinders or cartridges. There is excellent control of the freezing tip with no concern about overspray as there would be with liquid nitrogen sprays. It can be used in any direction and does not need to be held vertically above the lesion to be frozen. It is not as fast as liquid nitrogen spray and, as with the other above techniques, not as cold as liquid nitrogen, so it should not be used for the treatment of skin cancers. The unit needs to remain plugged in to maintain the chilling of the metal cores. The size and shape of the treatment area are constrained by the size and shape of the tips, but overlapping patterns can be used for irregular shapes. The refrigerator takes clinic space and there is a background noise that is added to the room in which it is stored.

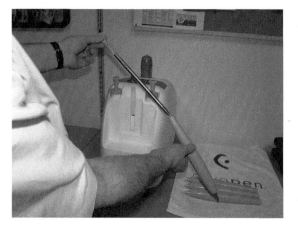

*Figure 4.8* Cryopen core, wands, and base unit. This is a refrigerant unit that remains plugged in to the wall for constant refrigeration of the wands. (Courtesy of Daniel Stulberg, MD.)

## CONCLUSION

There are multiple devices available that will achieve the desired temperatures for cryosurgery of benign conditions in the office-based setting. If a provider desires to treat skin cancers with cryosurgery, then they should choose the liquid nitrogen spray equipment. For the treatment of other skin lesions, all of the devices discussed above work very well. For a provider just starting with cryosurgery, he or she may wish to start with one of the disposable units because they have a lower start-up cost. They are also extremely portable and easy to store. For a provider who anticipates treating multiple patients over a long period of time, the units that have reusable components will typically have a lower per treatment cost. Access to liquid nitrogen and the ability to safely store it may deter some providers from using it. The tools discussed above are not dependent on routine delivery of liquid nitrogen. They may be ideal for a provider in a remote location or one who travels to multiple clinics because some are small enough to carry in a briefcase and based on their method of cooling can remain effective and ready to use even if stored for months or years.

## REFERENCE

1. Rowland AS, Baird DD, Weinberg CR, Shore DL, Shy CM, Wilcox AJ. Reduced fertility among women employed as dental assistants exposed to high levels of nitrous oxide. N Engl J Med. 1992 Oct 1;327(14): 993-7. PubMed PMID: 1298226.
2. Burkhart CG, Pchalek I, Adler M, Burkhart CN. An in vitro study comparing temperatures of over-the-counter wart preparations with liquid nitrogen. J Am Acad Dermatol 2007;57:1019–20.

# 5 Techniques

Safe and effective cryosurgery does not happen by chance. It requires a proper technique, which will vary according to the type and location of the lesion, and the equipment used. Chapter 3 deals with the equipment needed for liquid nitrogen treatment and Chapter 4 reviews the different apparatus needed for successful application of compressed gas, refrigerant liquids, and electrically cooled probes. This chapter deals with the practical techniques that allow the physician to use the various refrigerants in a clinical setting to effect safe and reproducible treatment of lesions. Important considerations include localization of the cryo-damage, with sparing of surrounding structures, ease of application, minimization of discomfort, and following protocols that are repeatable and reproducible within the limits of patient variability.

The cryosurgeon should bear in mind that skin comprises many constituent cell types, which have their own sensitivities to cryosurgery; these are listed in Table 5.1. Most notably, melanocytes are highly sensitive to freezing and this feature results in the clinical change of post-cryosurgical hypopigmentation. Connective tissue, on the other hand, is fairly resistant and this characteristic accounts for the maintenance of a structural framework in cryosurgery-treated tissue and thus limited contraction or hypertrophy. The cryosurgeon should also be mindful that the damage inflicted on the tissues is hugely dependent on the refrigerant, and the mode and duration of application of the treatment. Low temperatures can be very destructive to human skin and the treatment schedule should be devised appropriately so that neither excessive damage nor under-treatment results. The resting temperatures of

the different refrigerants are listed in Table 5.2. A strong understanding of the characteristics of the equipment, the cryogen, and the treatment techniques will lead to safe and effective cryosurgery.

## FREEZE TIME–THAW TIME

The freeze time is measured from the start of ice-ball formation to the end of the active freezing. This holds true whether the cryogen is sprayed on the skin or applied with a closed probe. The ice ball (also called icefield and freeze ball) is visible when the skin turns white. As it is not always easy to discern the start of the ice ball time, sometimes the freeze time is measured from the start of the freezing itself. This variability in definition and the lack of precision involved in determining the start of an ice ball mean that published freeze times must be considered as approximate guidelines rather than precision measurements. In practice few clinicians use a stopwatch to measure these times, so a lack of precise measurement is already inherent in the process.

Many cryosurgeons will freeze a lesion to the point that an ice ball covers all of the intended treatment area, and then start the counting that defines the freeze time. Unfortunately there are many different approaches to reaching that point. One operator may spray paint the area and achieve an overall (but superficial) ice ball quickly, whereas another may spray only in the center of the lesion (spot freeze) and allow the ice ball to gradually extend, creating a much deeper ice ball. The point at which they start counting the freeze time differs. Also, the use of cryoprobes tends to achieve an overall freeze at a different rate

Table 5.1  Relative Sensitivity to Low Temperatures

| Cells, tissues or organisms | Sensitivity |
| --- | --- |
| Melanocytes | Sensitive to cold injury (easily killed) |
| Basal cells | Less sensitive |
| Keratinocytes | ↓ |
| Bacteria | ↓ |
| Connective tissue | ↓ |
| Neural connective tissue sheath | ↓ |
| Vascular endothelium | ↓ |
| Viruses | Insensitive to cold injury |

Table 5.2  Temperatures of Cryogens

| Cryogens | Temperature (°C) |
| --- | --- |
| Ice | 0° |
| Ice/salt | −20° |
| Liquid nitrogen swab | −20° |
| Over-the-counter spray | −57° |
| Carbon dioxide cryogun | −70° |
| Refrigerant dispenser | −72° to −90° |
| Nitrous oxide cryogun | −89° |
| Nitrous oxide spray | −89° |
| Linear compression cryopen | −95° |
| Liquid nitrogen spray or probe | −196° |

to a spray. Where possible we have defined the method of application alongside the recommended freeze times to overcome some of these issues.

Thaw time is defined as the end of the active freezing (the spray has stopped or the probe is removed from the skin) until the ice ball is no longer visible. Although exact thaw times are rarely used to guide therapy, observing the approximate rate and time of a thaw can give additional information about the quality of the freeze performed, ie if the ice ball thaws faster than expected a second freeze–thaw cycle may be needed.

There are many variables that affect how the freeze time impacts the desired treatment. Although longer freeze times create more tissue destruction, the temperatures, depth, and internal shape of the freeze ball are also important treatment variables that are difficult to measure. The factors that can be controlled include the following:

- Open spray versus closed probe (or tweezer or cotton bud)
- Spray-tip aperture diameter
- Spray-tip configuration (straight versus bent)
- Distance to skin of the spray
- Spot freeze versus spray paint (or other pattern)
- Continuous versus intermittent spray (pulse)
- Impurities in liquid nitrogen (these can block the spray tip and cause an uneven spray)
- Level of liquid nitrogen in the spray gun.

These factors, in addition to the freeze time, will determine the temperatures within the ice ball, along with its depth, shape, and diameter. The expert cryosurgeon endeavors to control all of these factors to produce the optimal freeze. Tissue destruction is mostly a product of temperature and duration of the freeze. Measurement of temperatures with thermocouple needles in research settings has provided us with the initial data that inform cryosurgery. Access to infrared sensor technology on cryoguns provides more data on surface temperatures during cryosurgery for future clinical studies.

As current clinical studies provide freeze times and halo diameters to compare with clinical outcomes, we must guide our therapy with these parameters. However, a 10-second freeze time with one cryospray tip of one diameter or shape will not produce the same effect as a 10-second freeze time with a completely different spray tip. The distance to the skin affects the depth and shape of the ice ball, so that freeze time alone does not tell the whole story. A spot freeze will be colder in the center than the periphery, whereas a spray paint approach creates a more even cryogen application, with a broader flatter ice ball. Although the level of liquid nitrogen in the spray gun should not be an important parameter, in practice when the spray gun is nearly empty the rate of spray diminishes

before it quits. We hope not to have impurities in liquid nitrogen but in reality they do accumulate in the bottom of the Dewar tanks, and can be transferred into our spray guns. Impurities can be purged from the tank by emptying it before refilling. The use of filters in the fill tube and cryogun can also help keep the impurities out of the equation.

In the remainder of this chapter we discuss how to make choices to control these factors for optimal cryosurgery. Freeze times with liquid nitrogen are recommended in subsequent chapters, with the caveat that multiple variables are involved in each freeze beyond the time that can be measured.

## ICE-BALL GEOMETRY AND ISOTHERMS

A single spot freeze will create a hemispherically shaped ice ball. The depth and diameter can best be visualized with the gel pad (**Figure 5.1**). Unfortunately all we can see on the patient is the border of the freeze ball with no depth information. Note how the freeze ball geometry changes with different methods of liquid nitrogen application. Note how there is less lateral spread with the probe. Isotherms are the lines that can be drawn to link all points of equal temperature (**Figure 5.2**).

### Halo Diameter

Whatever method of cryosurgery is being used, it is crucial to understand the concept of the halo diameter. Most lesions will need to be frozen beyond the limit of their borders in order to destroy the whole lesion and not leave a rim of untreated tissue behind (**Figure 5.3**). The halo around the lesion is also called the peripheral zone of freezing. The halo diameter is just the length of this zone. Depending on the method of freeze, the freezing on the perimeter of the lesion usually does not get as cold as the center. Therefore, freezing beyond the border will provide sufficiently cold temperatures within the lesion for the desired destruction. This concept is referred to in all the remaining chapters because recommendations are made for the treatment of benign, premalignant, and malignant skin diseases. This is especially important for cryosurgery of malignant lesions, in which colder temperatures are needed and the risks of recurrence are accompanied by higher stakes.

For example, when planning cryosurgery for a basal cell carcinoma (BCC) it helps to consider that a surgical excision usually includes at least a 2- to 3-mm margin of normal skin. This margin can be drawn around the BCC and be referred to as margin X (**Figure 5.4**). Next, it must be remembered that freezing to margin X may achieve only a 0°C isotherm which is insufficient. The ice ball must be extended out another 2–3 mm so that the isotherm at margin X is now closer to −30°C. This extension beyond margin X becomes part of the halo diameter of 4–5 mm.

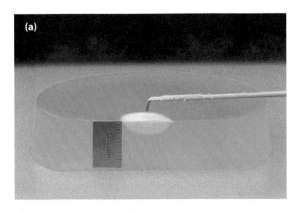

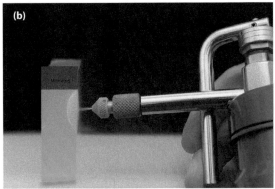

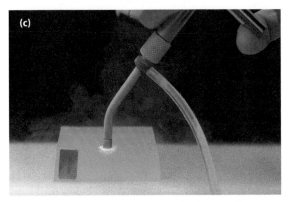

*Figure 5.1* (a) A single spot freeze for 60 seconds with liquid nitrogen and a bent spray extension. This has created a hemispherically shaped ice ball on an agar gel pad. The depth and diameter can be visualized. (b) Spot freeze for 60 seconds with a C tip has created a similar hemispherically shaped ice ball. (c) The ice-ball geometry is different when a probe is applied to the gel with 60 seconds of continuous freeze time. Note how there is less lateral spread with the probe. (Courtesy of Richard Usatine, MD.)

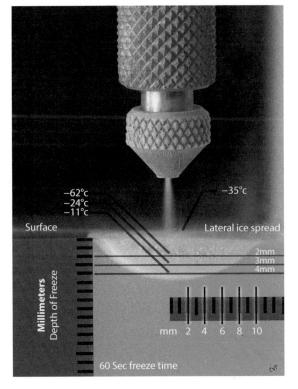

*Figure 5.2* An ice ball was produced by a spot freeze for 60 seconds using liquid nitrogen sprayed through a C tip onto an agar plate. The ice ball spreads out in a hemispherical pattern. Temperatures were measured using a thermocouple below the surface and infrared sensors from a Cry-Ac TrackerCam on the surface. The ice ball is coldest at the center just below the surface. Although the surface is receiving the cold spray it also is warmed by the ambient air above the agar, and the measured temperatures are somewhat colder just below the surface. In living tissue circulating blood warms the deeper parts so that the gradients are somewhat different. The coldest points of the ice ball are at the center, no matter the depth or model. (Courtesy of Richard Usatine, MD and Craig LaPlante.)

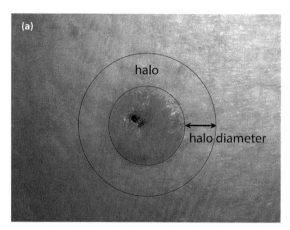 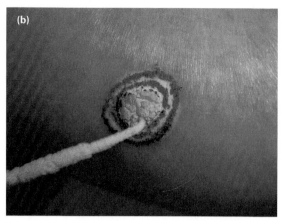

*Figure 5.3* (a) Halo diameter demonstrated around a nodular basal cell carcinoma on the back. Cryosurgery should include freezing out to the larger circle to ensure full destruction of the BCC. A shave biopsy would be performed to confirm the clinical diagnosis before treating with cryosurgery. (b) A halo with a 2 mm diameter was drawn around a common wart to obtain a lethal freeze at the edge of the wart. The freeze was performed with liquid nitrogen and a symmetric 360° halo around the wart was achieved. (Courtesy of Richard Usatine, MD.)

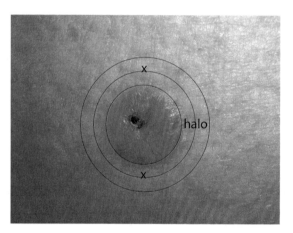

*Figure 5.4* When planning cryosurgery for a basal cell carcinoma (BCC) it helps to consider that a surgical excision usually includes at least a 2- to 3-mm margin of normal skin. This margin can be drawn around the BCC and be referred to as margin X. Next it must be remembered that freezing to margin X may achieve only a 0°C isotherm which is insufficient. The ice ball must be extended out another 2–3 mm so that the isotherm at margin X is now closer to −30°C. This extension beyond margin X becomes part of the halo diameter of 4–5 mm. A shave biopsy would be performed to confirm the clinical diagnosis before treating with cryosurgery. (Courtesy of Richard Usatine, MD.)

## LIQUID NITROGEN: COTTON SWAB TECHNIQUE

This is the simplest method for applying liquid nitrogen to skin lesions. It is used in office practice for the treatment of warts and other benign lesions. After decanting a small amount of liquid nitrogen into a suitable container (such as a Styrofoam cup), a cotton swab is dipped into the liquid and applied firmly to the lesion until a narrow halo of frozen tissue forms around it (**Figure 5.5**). When treating thin lesions such as actinic keratoses a 1-mm diameter of frozen peripheral tissue usually suffices. To achieve good results for thicker lesions, longer and more extensive peripheral freezes are needed, and it may be necessary to dip the swab into the liquid more than once before reapplying it to the skin. The duration of application will depend on the size and nature of the lesion to be treated but achievement of the peripheral frozen zone will remain the goal. Details of treatment for benign and premalignant lesions can be found in Chapters 8 and 9, respectively. This technique is not appropriate for malignant lesions because it is not sufficiently and predictably destructive for these high-risk lesions.

Cotton swabs are sometimes loosely bound whereas others are tightly bound; the latter will hold very little liquid nitrogen. The freezing impact of a large, loosely bound swab is many times that of a firm, small one and it is therefore impossible to write a protocol that could be universally adopted. Generally it is best to use a swab with a tip that is slightly smaller than the area to be treated. If necessary, tiny amounts of cotton can be wound around the tip of an orange stick to pinpoint the smallest skin lesions. Although it is safe to redip the swab several times into the receptacle for a given patient, the general view is that this should be discarded before treating another individual. Equally, the remnants from the receptacle should not be poured back into the main storage reservoir. This precaution is to prevent cross-contamination of the liquid nitrogen with human papillomaviruses, herpesviruses, and

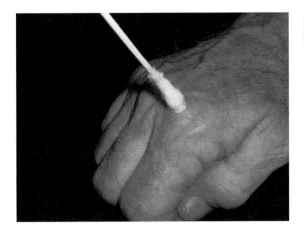

Figure 5.5 Cotton-wool bud application of liquid nitrogen to a common wart. Some additional cotton was added to a standard cotton-tipped applicator to increase the retention of liquid nitrogen. The ice ball formed can be seen extending onto normal skin by about 1 mm. (Courtesy of Richard Usatine, MD.)

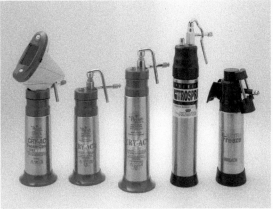

Figure 5.6 Multiple cryosurgical guns from Brymill, Premier, and Wallach. (Courtesy of Craig LaPlante.)

hepatitis viruses. Herpesviruses have been shown to survive temperatures as low as −196°C.[1]

Using the cotton swab technique, it is difficult to obtain temperatures below −20°C at depths greater than 2–3 mm. Therefore it is suitable only for relatively small superficial benign and premalignant skin lesions. It may take a little longer than some other techniques, but it is inexpensive for those with a supply of liquid nitrogen but no access to a cryogun.

## SPRAY TECHNIQUE

Several manufacturers produce spray guns which dispense liquid nitrogen. These guns enable the operator to treat many lesions on many patients before a refill is necessary (**Figure 5.6**). Manufacturers supply spray tips of various diameters and shapes to control the size and pattern of spray (see Figures 3.9–3.13, Chapter 3). The tips may be screwed on or attached via a Luer lock. The top of the spray gun is unscrewed and removed to allow filling via a fill tube or valve system. Once the top is screwed back on to the base of the spray gun, pressure develops inside and is released through the nozzle by pulling the trigger.

When the cryogun is about to be used, the tip should be held 1–2 cm away from the lesion and perpendicular to the skin (**Figure 5.7**). The gun should be held nearly upright to keep the gaseous phase in the upper portion of the gun and the liquid in the lower portion of the gun, where it is forced into the tube that directs the liquid nitrogen spray through the nozzle. The target lesion must be clearly identified in order to achieve the correct peripheral zone of freezing (halo). It is sometimes helpful to mark the desired margins of freeze around the lesion, especially

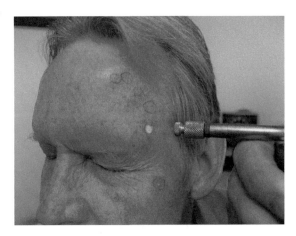

Figure 5.7 Cryosurgery performed with cryospray from a cryogun held 1–2 cm from actinic keratoses, which were marked with a ballpoint pen before cryosurgery.

when first starting out doing cryosurgery, with irregularly shaped lesions and difficult-to-see lesions such as actinic keratoses that are detected by palpation. A surgical marking pen can be used, but a ballpoint pen may also be used, the ink being easily removed with an alcohol swab. Although actinic keratoses are often better felt than seen, the application of liquid nitrogen often makes the borders more visible.

## SPOT FREEZE VERSUS OTHER PATTERNS
## OF FREEZE

For small lesions, the spray should be directed at the middle of the lesion until the desired diameter of freeze is achieved. This is called a spot freeze (see Figure 5.2). If the diameter of freeze is spreading out too quickly or the clinician desires a deeper depth of freeze for the diameter,

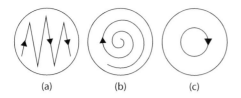

*Figure 5.8* Various liquid nitrogen spray directional techniques used to provide even ice production within the defined treatment field: (a) spray paint; (b) spiral; (c) rotary.

the trigger can be pulsed to provide an intermittent spray, allowing for deeper tissue penetration. For larger superficial lesions (such as a large seborrheic keratosis), a spray paint, spiral, or rotary technique is used to freeze a broad area of tissue without freezing the deeper tissues (**Figure 5.8**). Of course, if the spray paint technique is continued for at least 30 seconds a deeper freeze may be obtained (this technique is used for superficial BCCs over 2 cm in diameter).

The spot-freeze method is only satisfactory for the cryosurgical treatment of lesions up to about 1.5 cm in diameter. Beyond this size, tissue temperatures at the periphery only reach −15°C and may be insufficient to achieve the desired destructive effect. This may leave an outside ring of untreated disease and risk the recurrence of malignant lesions. For lesions larger than 1.5 cm in diameter, the area may be treated with overlapping circles of spot freezes. We prefer the spray paint, spiral, or rotary techniques (Figure 5.8) applied evenly and long enough to achieve the desired depth of freeze across the entire lesion.

Colder temperatures may be attainable with a double freeze–thaw cycle because the tissue remains colder after the first thaw is over. This is demonstrated in **Figure 5.9** with two 30-second freeze times. The colder temperatures are found at the shallower depths but −60°C is still reached at 6 mm depth in the second freeze.

### CONTINUOUS SPRAY VERSUS INTERMITTENT PULSE SPRAY

Cryospray can be delivered as a continuous spray or with intermittent pulses. A spot freeze with a continuous spray may be appropriate for some lesions. However, when the desired halo diameter is about to be surpassed with the continuous spray, the freeze time can be prolonged with intermittent pulses of spray while keeping the spray within the desired halo diameter (**Figure 5.10**). Figure 5.8 provides diagrams to understand how the pattern of spray can affect the depth of treatment.

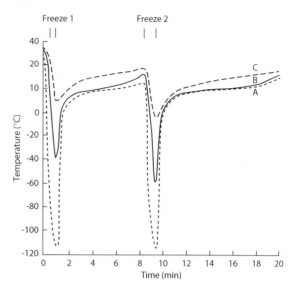

*Figure 5.9* Temperatures recorded using thermocouple technology during a double freeze–thaw cycle with liquid nitrogen spray for 30 seconds after ice-ball formation. The spot-freeze method was used and temperatures were measured at 2-mm depth (curve A), 6-mm depth (curve B), and 10-mm depth (curve C). Note how the temperatures become colder during the second freeze which started at a colder temperature.

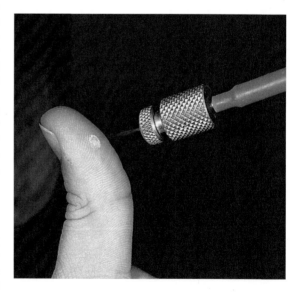

*Figure 5.10* An intermittent pulsatile spray was used to constrain the pattern of liquid nitrogen spread while treating a small wart with a C-tip aperture. (Courtesy of Usatine R, Moy R, Tobinick E, Siegel D. Skin Surgery: A practical guide. St. Louis, MO: Mosby, 1998.)

## SPRAY TIPS FOR LIQUID NITROGEN

As discussed in Chapter 3, there are several spray tips for the various cryoguns that have different aperture diameters and shapes for specific purposes. In most clinical situations, the brass C tip for the Brymill unit is very useful (see Figure 5.2). The straight spray extensions can be useful for treating small skin lesions and the higher-end units with infrared sensing and video attachments utilize the spray extension to achieve the right distance for sensing and cryosurgery at the same time (**Figure 5.11**). A bent spray extension tip is useful to reach less accessible skin lesions as well as mucosal lesions in the mouth and vagina. This tip can also be rotated to spray in any direction that is useful, and at times it is easier to adjust the direction of spray rather than the position of the patient.

The bent spray tip attenuates the flow of the liquid nitrogen so that the spray is less shocking to the patient. It is optimal for the following:

- Children and adults who fear this therapy – warts and molluscum (**Figure 5.12**)
- Pinpoint accuracy on smaller lesions – molluscum and small warts (**Figure 5.13**)
- Faces and noses which are sensitive to pain – great for actinic keratoses (**Figure 5.14**)
- Condyloma on genitalia to minimize pain (**Figure 5.15**).

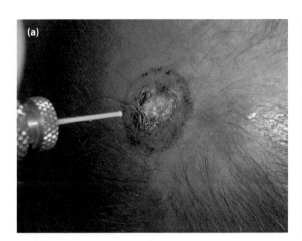

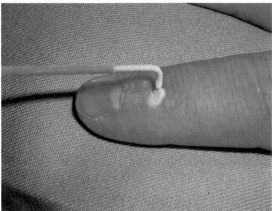

*Figure 5.12* Bent spray extension used to treat warts on the fingers of a young child. The slow attenuated spray makes this method less painful and scary for young children. (Courtesy of Richard Usatine, MD.)

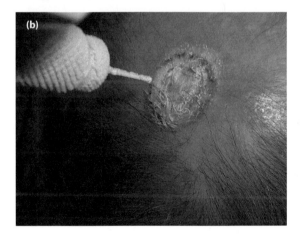

*Figure 5.11* Cryospray with liquid nitrogen being delivered through a straight extension for the treatment of a basal cell carcinoma on the scalp. (a) The spot-freeze method is being used and the green light represents a temperature of below 0°C measured by infrared sensing technology. (b) The light was set to turn red at a temperature below −30°C. Note how the halo diameter was drawn on the skin and the freeze was maintained until the full halo was frozen. (Courtesy of Richard Usatine, MD.)

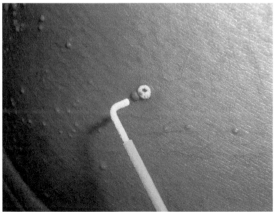

*Figure 5.13* Bent spray extension used to treat small molluscum lesions in the pubic area. The slow attenuated spray is optimal for small lesions in general. (Courtesy of Richard Usatine, MD.)

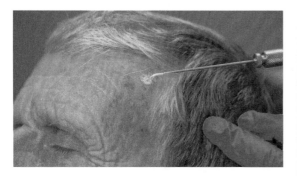

*Figure 5.14* Bent spray extension used to treat actinic keratosis on the face. The slow attenuated spray is more comfortable on the face and easy to control for actinic keratoses. (Courtesy of Richard Usatine, MD.)

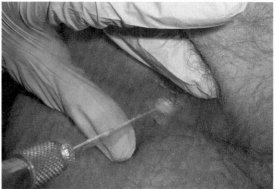

*Figure 5.16* The long straight extension spray is optimal for perianal condyloma. (Courtesy of Richard Usatine, MD.)

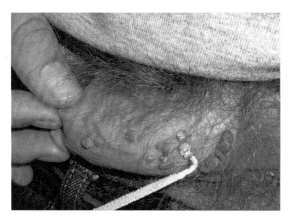

*Figure 5.15* Bent spray extension used to treat condyloma on the penis. The slow attenuated spray is less shocking to the patient and easy to control for small condyloma. (Courtesy of Richard Usatine, MD.)

The long, straight, spray-needle extension is helpful when treating condyloma in the anogenital regions (**Figure 5.16**). The length delivers the liquid nitrogen into these areas while keeping the cryogun and clinician at a healthy distance.

### Constraining the Spray

The easiest way to constrain the spray is to use small aperture tips, bent spray extensions, and an intermittent spray when needed. It is often helpful to localize the spray's area of skin contact especially when working close to sensitive areas such as the eyes. Spray shields, cones, and simple improvised barriers can prevent overspray or concentrate the spray to a focused area. There are commercially available neoprene cones and a clear plastic disc with four different diameter openings that can be used to constrain the liquid nitrogen spray (see Figures 3.17–3.19, Chapter 3). Otoscope tips can also be used. For cryosurgery

near the eye or other sensitive structures, overspray can be prevented by using a tongue depressor, gauze, or a tongue depressor wrapped with gauze (**Figure 5.17**).

Adhesive putty may be used to create custom-fitted spray shields. This is helpful for irregularly shaped lesions or for freezing skin cancers to help constrain the spray because skin cancers require much more aggressive freezing than benign lesions (**Figure 5.18**). Chapter 10 discusses cryosurgery of skin cancers in detail.

### LIQUID NITROGEN-ADHERENT PROBES (CRYOPROBES)

Liquid nitrogen spray guns can be fitted with adherent probes instead of spray tips. A solid metal tip is chilled by the flow of liquid nitrogen, which is then vented off through a flexible plastic tube (**Figures 5.19 and 5.20**). This is especially useful for vascular lesions such as venous lakes and hemangiomas. The solid probe tip is used to compress the lesion, emptying some of the contents, so that the volume is reduced. When the device is activated producing a visible icefield, the cold effect reaches deeper into the tissue when pressure is applied (Figure 5.20).

The treatment of the following lesions may benefit from the cryoprobe most (see Chapter 8 for more details on the treatment of all these benign lesions):

- Angiofibromas
- Angiomas (cherry and spider)
- Digital mucus cysts (Figure 5.19)
- Hemangiomas (Figure 5.20)
- Lymphangiomas
- Mucoceles
- Pyogenic granulomas
- Venous lakes.

Various probe sizes are available, with the smallest being suitable for spider angiomas and lesions in sensitive areas (where it may be awkward to use a spray tip) and

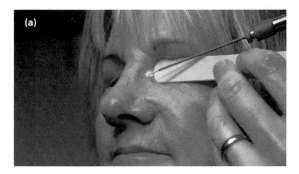

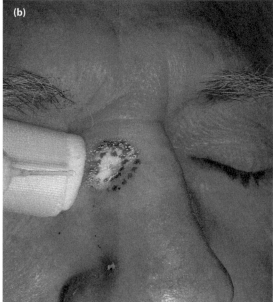

*Figure 5.17* (a) A tongue depressor is being used to protect the eye from liquid nitrogen spray in the treatment of a seborrheic keratosis. (b) A tongue depressor wrapped with cotton gauze is a great eye protector for the longer freeze time needed to treat a basal cell carcinoma near the eye. (Courtesy of Richard Usatine, MD.)

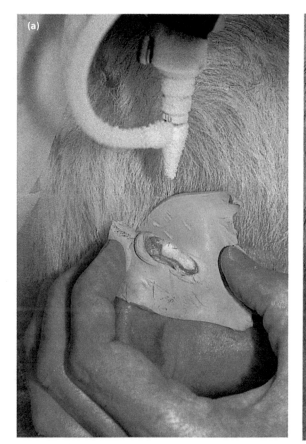

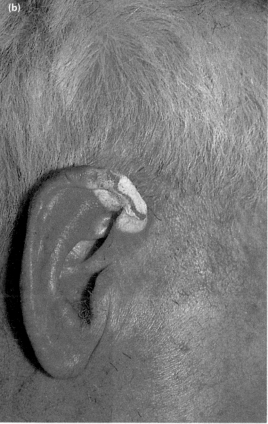

*Figure 5.18* (a) Adhesive putty – an appropriately sized piece has been chosen to surround the field to be treated on the ear. (b) The icefield has been induced and the putty removed.

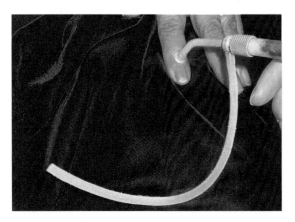

*Figure 5.19* Cryoprobe frozen with liquid nitrogen is applied to a digital mucus cyst to freeze the base of the cyst after it has been drained with a needle. Note how the plastic ventilation tube is pointing away from the patient's hand. (Courtesy of Richard Usatine, MD.)

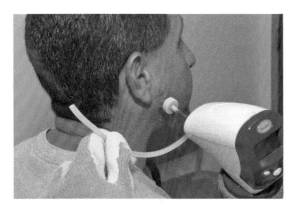

*Figure 5.20* Compressing and freezing a hemangioma with a cryoprobe. Note how the plastic ventilation tube is being held away from the patient's skin in the protected gloved hand. The cryoprobe was made cold before contact with the skin to avoid sticking to the skin. (Courtesy of Richard Usatine, MD).

the wider probes for large and deeper-seated hemangiomas. Care must be taken not to create unwanted damage because there is a tendency for the probe to adhere to the tissue at the end of the treatment and continue to exert its destructive effect. This can be avoided by freezing the probe first and then applying it to the skin, and continuing to run liquid nitrogen through the probe. Alternately, a small amount of water-soluble gel at the interface will facilitate the freezing process but also allows the probe to release more quickly from the skin.

Care is needed to ensure that the nitrogen that is venting through the ventilation tube does not come into contact with the patient. The flexible tubes may wave about until they become frozen by the nitrogen passing through. Once the tube is frozen it will stay in place and the spray should be unidirectional away from the patient (see Figure 5.19). Adherent probe tips should be wiped down with standard alcohol wipes and not bleach (alcohol for cleaning is recommended by the manufacturer). See Box 5.1 for pearls in the use of liquid nitrogen probes.

### FORCEPS (CRYO TWEEZERS)
The use of Cryo Tweezers is a great technique for the following lesions:

- Skin tags
- Warts and skin tags on the eyelids (**Figure 5.21**)
- Filiform warts in children (**Figure 5.22**).

---

*Box 5.1* Pearls for Liquid Nitrogen Probes

- Freeze the end of the probe before applying it to the patient to avoid the probe sticking to the patient.
- If the probe sticks to the patient, do not pull it off because significant tissue damage may occur. If the probe is taking longer than expected to detach from the patient use your fingers or warm water to rewarm the adherent probe.
- If you do not have a probe equal to the size of the lesion, it is better to choose a smaller one and freeze longer than to use a larger probe which will unnecessarily destroy normal surrounding tissue.

---

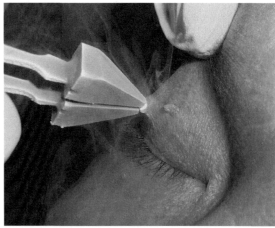

*Figure 5.21* Cryo Tweezers being used to freeze pedunculated skin tags on the upper eyelid. This is a safe and relatively painless method of treating pedunculated benign lesions on the eyelids. (Courtesy of Richard Usatine, MD.)

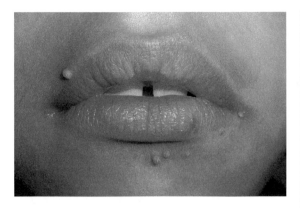

*Figure 5.22* Multiple filiform warts around the mouth of an 8-year-old boy after treatment with Cryo Tweezers. A common wart on the same child's finger was treated with cryospray. The child found the Cryo Tweezers to be much less painful. (Courtesy of Richard Usatine, MD.)

The skin tags are grasped and held with the Cryo Tweezers until the freeze margin reaches the normal tissue at the skin surface. The tweezers can be used to treat many more skin tags before they warm up. Re-immerse the tweezers in the liquid nitrogen when you note that the freeze time is lengthening. The Cryo Tweezers are particularly good for skin tags or warts on the eyelids. After grasping the elevated papule pull the whole lid away from the eye to protect the globe from cryodamage (Figure 5.20). Then continue the freeze until the whole tag or wart is white to the base. This avoids any spray that may enter the eye. It also results in less unnecessary overtreatment of the surrounding skin by overspray (**Figure 5.23**). Cryo Tweezers can be cleaned between patients by allowing them to reach room temperature, and wiping with an alcohol wipe. Some clinicians use standard surgical forceps or heavy hemostats, but these do not retain the cold as long and require frequent redipping in the liquid nitrogen.

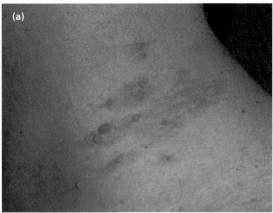
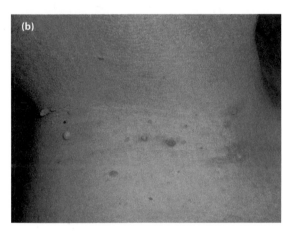

*Figure 5.23* Skin tags on the neck of one patient were treated with liquid nitrogen using cryospray on one side and Cryo Tweezers on the other side. (a) Cryospray of left neck showing significant erythema around the skin tags from overspray. (b) Cryo Tweezers treatment of right neck showing very little erythema surrounding the skin tags because the treatment is more precise. (Courtesy of Richard Usatine, MD.)

### MULTIPLE FREEZE–THAW CYCLES
Especially when treating thicker lesions or skin cancers, it is helpful to allow the icefield to thaw before applying a second period of freezing. The second freeze does increase cell destruction and one study supports the double freeze for basal cell carcinomas on the face.[2] Some studies have shown better clinical results by employing this technique, especially with the treatment of plantar warts.[3] The thawing phase will usually take three to four times the duration of the freeze. Once the lesion is no longer visibly or palpably frozen, the second freeze is performed. If the thaw time is shorter than expected, this is a good reason to do a second freeze because this may make up for an inadequately short initial freeze. For this reason, it is helpful not only to look at freeze times but also to watch the rate and duration of the thaw time. The second freeze usually starts more quickly but should be maintained for the desired time of freeze or diameter of freeze margin (Figure 5.9).

Chapters 8–10 provide details of freezing schedules using liquid nitrogen for benign, premalignant, and malignant skin lesions.

## COMPRESSED GAS CRYOGUNS

The cryogun is attached to the gas cylinder (usually nitrous oxide) via a flexible tube and an adapter that screws onto the cylinder (**Figure 5.24**). Carbon dioxide can be used but is slower and the cryoguns cannot be interchanged between the two gases without refitting them. It is important to make sure that gaskets are in good repair and the unit is carefully threaded onto the gas cylinder to prevent leaking. Opening the valve of the gas cylinder allows the clinician to check if there is adequate pressure for cryosurgery. Most of the gauges will read a green or blue optimal range. If the pressure is higher than the acceptable range for the cryosurgery unit, the adapter should be removed from the gas cylinder and some of the gas should be released from the cylinder in a safe, well-ventilated location. The clinician should use caution because the release of the excess gas is extremely loud. The adapter is then reattached to the gas cylinder to make sure that the pressure is in the safe operating range.

There are a variety of exchangeable tips in different shapes and sizes that can be screwed on to the cryogun (**Figure 5.25**). For cryosurgery of the skin, a 1-mm tip is useful for fine work, including small warts or skin tags. A 3- to 4-mm rounded or beveled tip is useful for larger warts, seborrheic keratoses, and other medium-sized lesions. There are larger disk-shaped tips that are used in cryosurgery for the treatment of cervical dysplasia. Occasionally these can be useful in cryosurgery of large skin lesions, but it should be noted that distinct circular areas of hypopigmentation will result from the use of these large round disks. To avoid discrete geometric shapes, they can be partially touched to the affected areas or overlapped for very broad areas.

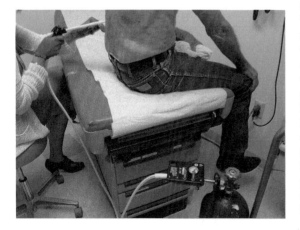

*Figure 5.24* Nitrous oxide cryogun with flexible tubing attached to storage cylinder being used to freeze seborrheic keratoses on the back. (Courtesy of Daniel Stulberg, MD.)

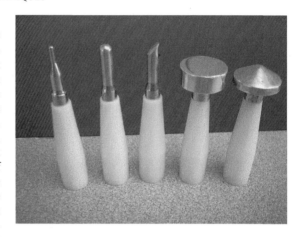

*Figure 5.25* Various tips for nitrous oxide and carbon dioxide cryoguns. The smaller tips are more appropriate for the skin and the larger tips were designed for the cervix. (Courtesy of Daniel Stulberg, MD.)

Once the appropriate tip has been selected, it should be dipped in a water-soluble gel and then touched to the lesion before activation of the unit. The water-soluble gel will facilitate the transmission of the cold temperature to the lesion and also help in release of the cryoprobe. After the tip is in contact with the skin, the clinician presses the activating trigger to allow the release of the compressed gas. The cold temperature is then transmitted to the tip of the cryogun and the water-soluble gel will start to freeze; as the skin freezes the probe will actually adhere to the skin. At this point the clinician can gently lift up the probe, which will tent the skin upward (**Figure 5.26**). This may reduce the damage to underlying subcutaneous structures. Once the desired diameter of freeze has been achieved around the skin lesion, the trigger is released to stop the active freeze. Table 5.3 gives some recommended freeze diameters. Most units have a quick-release/quick-thaw function that is activated by a separate button or by a quick pull of the trigger, causing release of the stored gas in the unit. The cryoprobe will then release from the skin and the frozen water-soluble gel. After thawing, a repeat freeze cycle can be performed if desired, based on the type of lesion. If there are multiple lesions to be treated, the clinician can dip the tip into the water-soluble gel and apply it to multiple lesions before freezing each individual lesion. Once cryosurgery has been completed the water-soluble gel is wiped from the patient's skin. The cryosurgery tip should be wiped down with appropriate bactericidal/virucidal solutions such as bleach-based disposable wipes.

## COMPRESSED-GAS DIRECT SPRAY DEVICES

To activate the Cryomega disposable unit, a lever-type device which comes in the extended position is folded into the main unit, unsealing the cartridge. This lever also

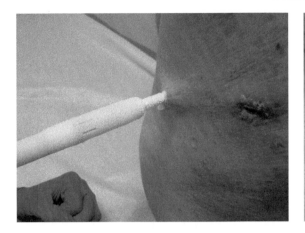

Figure 5.26 Tenting the skin up after the freeze has caused adherence of the probe to the skin. (Courtesy of Daniel Stulberg, MD.)

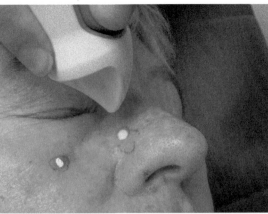

Figure 5.27 Treatment of multiple actinic keratoses with Cryomega disposable nitrous oxide spray unit. Note the continued ice ball on the actinic keratosis previously treated on the cheek. (Courtesy of Daniel Stulberg, MD.)

Table 5.3 Recommended Halo Diameters for Nitrous Oxide Cryoguns

| Lesion | Margin of freeze beyond the lesion |
|---|---|
| Lentigines | 1 mm single freeze |
| Actinic keratoses | 1 mm freeze, thaw, freeze |
| Seborrheic keratoses | 2 mm freeze, thaw, freeze |
| Plantar and common warts | 3 mm freeze, thaw, freeze |

becomes the trigger for the unit, which can be used for multiple lesions and even at different clinical sessions until the cartridge is empty (**Figure 5.27**). The reusable cryoprobe device has three different-sized tips that can be unscrewed and changed out based on the size of the desired spray for smaller or larger lesions. To activate the unit, a filter is placed in the distal half of the unit and a new nitrous oxide cartridge is placed against it, with the closed portion of the cartridge aligned in the proximal portion of the cylindrical unit. The seal of the cartridge is pierced by a quick twisting closure of the two halves of the unit. Remove the cap from one of the desired tips and depress the trigger on the side of the unit to spray the desired lesions. With either the disposable or the reusable devices, hold the unit 0.5–1 cm vertically above the lesions for the desired freeze time (**Figure 5.28**). Raising the device will cause a broader spray; lowering it will focus the spray as needed to the lesion size. The remainder of the gas in the cartridge can be used at another session, but over time does tend to bleed off, and when needed a new cartridge is inserted (see Table 5.4 for some recommended freeze times).

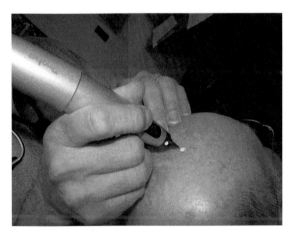

Figure 5.28 Using the cryoprobe reusable nitrous oxide spray to freeze actinic keratosis. (Courtesy of Daniel Stulberg, MD.)

Table 5.4 Recommended Freeze Times for Cryoprobe Nitrous Oxide Spray (per manufacturer)

| Lesion | Freeze time |
|---|---|
| Lentigines | 6 seconds single freeze |
| Cherry angiomas | 10 seconds single freeze |
| Actinic keratoses | 10 seconds freeze, thaw, freeze |
| Sebaceous hyperplasia | 10 seconds freeze, thaw, freeze |
| Warts | 5 seconds per millimeter of wart depth |

## REFRIGERANT LIQUIDS

There are two methods of using refrigerant liquids. The first involves constraining the liquid to a specific area and allowing it to evaporate off to effect a freeze. The clinician selects an appropriate size plastic cone provided with the unit (or alternate devices are available) that surrounds the lesion to be treated. The refrigerant liquid is sprayed into the cone while it is firmly pressed against the skin to make a liquid-tight seal (**Figure 5.29**). After 3.2–6.4 mm (eighth to a quarter of an inch) of liquid is present at the bottom of the cone, the clinician stops the spray and allows the liquid to evaporate before lifting the cone from the skin. When the cone is lifted it will reveal the frozen tissue in a circular pattern that was covered by the cone (Figure 5.29). Lifting the cone too soon or not applying it firmly enough to the skin will allow the refrigerant liquid to run off, giving an inadequate freeze to the lesion and often a superficial freeze of the runoff area. Different sized lesions can be treated with the various cone tips or the use of a commercially available plastic disk that has four different cone sizes (see Figure 3.17, Chapter 3). This is the same device that is used to prevent overspray with liquid nitrogen spray techniques.

The second method of freezing with refrigerant liquids is to use them in the same method as a cotton swab dipped in liquid nitrogen. The refrigerant liquid can be sprayed directly on the swabs that come with the product and then touched to the lesion to be frozen (**Figure 5.30**). Some of the refrigerant liquid products come with swabs that consist of a hollow tube which can be inserted into the tip of the canister. The refrigerant liquid is sprayed through the tube into the foam distal portion of the swab. Once the liquid stops dripping from the foam swab, it can then be touched to the lesion to perform cryosurgery (**Figure 5.31**). (See Table 5.5 for some recommended freeze times.)

## ELECTRICAL REFRIGERATION

The desktop electrical refrigeration unit is typically plugged into a standard wall outlet in the office to maintain the unit at the appropriate temperature (**Figure 5.32**).

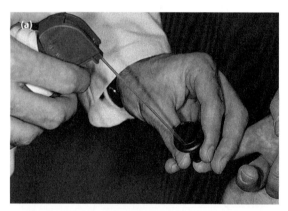

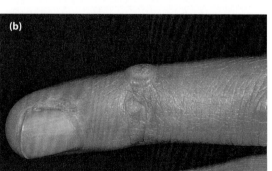

*Figure 5.29* (a) The liquid cryogen (verruca freeze) is being sprayed into a cone, slightly larger than the wart, pressed firmly against the skin. (b) Blister formed around wart after using evaporative technique with a restraining cone. (Courtesy of Usatine R, Moy R, Tobinick E, Siegel D. Skin Surgery: A practical guide. St. Louis, MO: Mosby, 1998.)

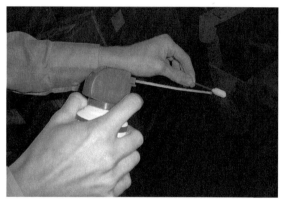

*Figure 5.30* Spraying liquid refrigerant onto a swab to use for cryosurgery. (Courtesy of Daniel Stulberg, MD.)

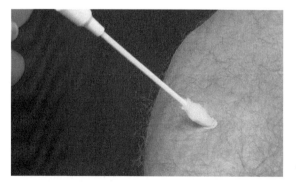

*Figure 5.31* Freezing with the cooled swab of the Histofreezer. (Courtesy of Daniel Stulberg, MD.)

*Table 5.5* Recommended Freeze Times for Verruca-Freeze Refrigerant Liquid (per manufacturer)

| Lesion | Freeze time (s) |
|---|---|
| Molluscum contagiosum | 20 |
| Lentigines | 25–35 |
| Verruca plana | 20–30 |
| Genital lesions | 20–30 |
| Actinic keratoses | 20–35 |
| Skin tags | 25–35 |
| Seborrheic keratoses | 30–40 |
| Verruca vulgaris | 30–40 |
| Verruca plantaris | 40 |

Freeze–thaw–freeze recommended for lesions >5 mm, deep or difficult lesions (eg plantar warts).

pattern of applications can be used. Check to see if the core is appropriately chilled by pressing the testing device firmly on top of the core in the unit. Green indicates that it is cold enough to proceed (Figure 5.32). The metal core is removed from the refrigeration unit and placed into the plastic wand-type handle with the attached metal probe (**Figure 5.34**). The probe is then touched to the lesion until the desired diameter of freeze is obtained (**Figure 5.35**). If there are multiple lesions and the rate of freezing slows down, the metal core is reinserted into the chilling unit after dipping in the supplied alcohol solution, and another previously cooled core is inserted into the probe to continue performing cryosurgery. The manufacturer recommends that the aluminum tips be cleaned with alcohol between patient usage and that agents containing bleach be avoided. Box 5.2 gives advice on the liquid nitrogen spray technique.

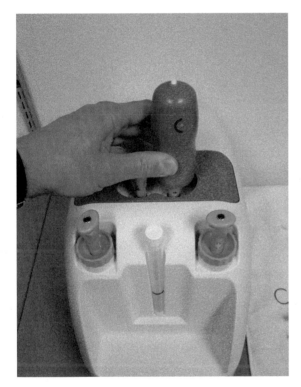

*Figure 5.32* Cryopen base unit is a refrigeration unit that is plugged into a wall socket. The green light indicates the probe is the correct temperature for cryosurgery. (Courtesy of Daniel Stulberg, MD.)

This assures that the device is ready when the need arises for cryosurgery. The clinician selects an appropriate size tip based on the size of the lesion (**Figure 5.33**). The tip size should approximate the diameter of the lesion. For lesions larger than the available tip sizes, an overlapping

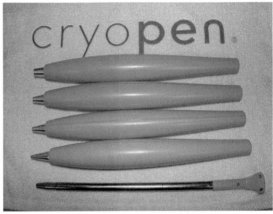

*Figure 5.33* Cryopen core and skin probes with different size tips. (Courtesy of Daniel Stulberg, MD.)

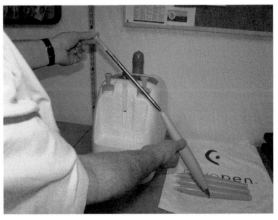

*Figure 5.34* Inserting chilled cryopen core into probe. (Courtesy of Daniel Stulberg, MD.)

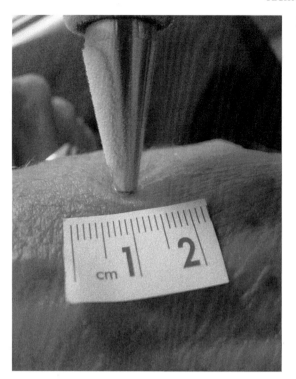

*Figure 5.35* Freezing a wart with the cryopen. (Courtesy of Daniel Stulberg, MD.)

REFERENCES

1. Burke WA, Baden TJ, Wheeler CE, Bowdre JH. Survival of herpes simplex virus during cryosurgery with liquid nitrogen. J Dermatol Surg Oncol 1986;12:1033–5.
2. Mallon E, Dawber R. Cryosurgery in the treatment of basal cell carcinoma. Assessment of one and two freeze-thaw cycle schedules. Dermatol Surg 1996;22:854–58.
3. Kwok CS, Gibbs S, Bennett C, et al. Topical treatments for cutaneous warts. Cochrane Database Syst Rev 2012;9:CD001781.

---

*Box 5.2* Ten Pearls for Liquid Nitrogen Spray Technique

1. Hold the cryogun relatively upright to avoid having the liquid $N_2$ come out of the valve and scare everyone in the room.
2. Make sure that the patient is in a stable position and not a moving target. If the lesion is on the hand, see that the hand is resting on the patient or furniture so that it doesn't move.
3. Hold the tip 1–2 cm from the lesion making sure that the spray is perpendicular to the skin. If using a bent spray probe, adjust the position of the cryogun and tip to achieve the 90° angle. Stabilize your hands and body so that your aim will be accurate and consistent.
4. Compress the trigger to start the spray. The pattern of spray should be determined by the size, elevation and depth of the lesion. The following techniques are options:
   - Steady continuous spray will produce wider shallow freeze zone. This may be sufficient for actinic keratoses and benign lesions.
   - Pulsing the spray intermittently in one spot will cause the freeze to stay localized (less lateral spread) and deepen with the duration of spray. This is good for thicker lesions such as common warts, molluscum, dermatofibromas, and keloids.
   - Using a spray paint technique of moving the spray in a back-and-forth motion will give a more superficial freeze for superficial lesions, including actinic keratoses and lentigines. Moving the spray back and forth across the lip may be sufficient for actinic cheilitis.
5. If you have the Cry-Ac TrackerCam pay attention to the tissue temperature and use this as one extra data point to guide your treatments.
6. Make sure that the freeze reaches all edges of the lesion with the desired halo diameter. The halo should be symmetrical around the lesion. It may be necessary to move the spray slightly back and forth to achieve an oval or linear pattern rather than a circle.
7. Freeze times vary based not on the diagnosis alone; smaller thinner lesions should receive less freeze time than larger thicker lesions even when the diagnosis is the same.
8. Watch the thawing. If the area thaws asymmetrically it may mean that one area did not get sufficient freeze time. You can add some freezing to that area. If the whole area thaws faster than expected, consider a second freeze–thaw cycle.
9. If the lesion is hypertrophic (especially with warts) consider paring it down with a scalpel or razor blade so that the base can be more effectively treated.
10. If you will be treating a lesion for more than 25 seconds give the patient a choice to have a local anesthetic first. Especially if treating a malignancy with two 30-second freezes, then lidocaine can be very helpful.

# 6 Preparation, consent, documentation, and aftercare

## TRAINING

Trainees in the specialties that regularly use cryosurgical methods should receive teaching and training on all aspects of the subject and be observed carrying out treatments. Hands-on workshops are a great way to augment training received or to get an introduction to cryosurgery. Good workshops will demonstrate the use of cryosurgical equipment and provide practical hands-on instruction using gel blocks, bananas, pigs' feet, or other models. Cryosurgical science and safety information should be provided. An alternative is to "sit in" with an experienced cryosurgeon on several occasions to see the skills, the range of suitable pathologies, and the approach to the patient. Beginners should gain significant personal experience in treating benign lesions before progressing to the treatment of malignant lesions. See Appendix B for information on learning methods. Of course, the text and images of this book provide much of the cognitive information needed to learn the art and science of cryosurgery.

## CRYOSURGERY ENVIRONMENT

Both the physician and patient must be adequately prepared for a cryosurgical procedure. It is best to perform procedures in well-lit, aerated rooms with a procedural chair/exam table/couch available for patients to lie down should they feel unwell or faint. Some procedures may take place as part of the initial consultation. In other situations patients will be asked to come back for an appointment set aside for cryosurgery, having had time to consider the therapeutic options. Among the pieces of equipment needed are the cryogen, delivery system, consent forms, blades to pare down excess keratin, and post-treatment dressings.

If a biopsy has been taken previously to ascertain the diagnosis, the report should be available before treatment. A short series of questions, with regard to specific health issues, should allow the physician to be sure that there are no contraindications to treatment. It is not essential to have an assistant present for minor freezing procedures. However, for larger lesions, when monitoring is being used and a patient is apprehensive, a medical assistant can play a crucial role. The assistant may help to prepare the patient, assist during the procedure, and have a role in further communication, reassurance, and wound care advice after the event.

## CONSENT

Patients should be properly informed about the treatment options for their condition, the relative merits of each and the side effects and complications of the treatment chosen (see consent form in Box 6.1). There is no consensus on whether or how the consent to treatment should be documented. Some organizations are satisfied with a verbal consent or a written summary of the discussion whereas others require the patient's signature at the end of a detailed document. In the case of simple procedures such as cryosurgery it is reasonable, and usually expected by the patient, to proceed immediately with treatment.

It is not surprising that claims are made against doctors after cryosurgery if no warning has been given of the potential side effects. Consider the treatment of viral warts on the fingers – blisters may appear as a result of treatment, which may not unduly bother a young teenager but may cause difficulty working for people in manual occupations. Informed consent for a cryosurgical procedure, whether a separate document that the patient signs or part of the clinician's case notes, should include discussion of the following points:

- Method of delivery of the refrigerant
- Condition to be treated (with expected results)
- Possible side effects, eg swelling, blisters
- Probable cosmetic outcome.

The need for an in-depth discussion is more relevant for more aggressive freeze protocols, when treating malignant disease, and when dealing with cosmetically or functionally important anatomical sites.

An example of a patient education handout on cryosurgery aftercare is found in Box 6.3.

## USE OF ANESTHESIA

All patients feel some degree of discomfort when their skin is subjected to ultra-low temperatures. The subjectivity of pain means that this varies enormously from patient to patient. Some individuals tolerate multiple, prolonged, freeze–thaw cycle methods whereas others will be upset by short freezes. Even the shortest cotton-bud freezes cause a perceptible "burning" or "stinging" sensation. Prolonged freeze times and those methods involving rapid lowering of temperature cause more pain. Immediate pain is felt by the superficial nerve endings before the anesthetic effect of freezing has time to act. Pain during the thaw phase, particularly after "tumor dose" methods, may last for many minutes and be profound if anesthesia was not used.

Certain anatomic sites are more likely to produce pain – particularly fingers, pulp and periungual area, ear, lips, temples, and the scalp. Even though this pain is usually

*Box 6.1* Disclosure and Consent Cryosurgery

**TO THE PATIENT:** You have the right, as a patient, to be informed about your condition and the recommended cryosurgical procedure to be used so that you may make the decision whether or not to undergo the procedure after knowing the risks and hazards involved. There are many benefits to cryosurgery including the eradication of the skin condition to be treated. This disclosure is not meant to scare or alarm you; it is simply an effort to make you better informed so you may give or withhold your informed consent to the procedure.

**I (we)** voluntarily request Dr. _____  _____
as my physician, and such associates, technical assistants and other healthcare providers as they may deem necessary to treat my condition which has been explained to me as _____
_____.

**I (we)** voluntarily consent and authorize cryosurgery.

Just as there may be risks and hazards in continuing my present condition without treatment, there are also risks and hazards related to the cryosurgery. **I (we)** also realize that the following risks and hazards may occur:

**PAIN, SWELLING, BLISTERS, CHANGE IN PIGMENTATION IN THE TREATED AREA, SLOW HEALING, BLEEDING, INFECTION, SCARRING, RE-GROWTH, CHANGE IN ANATOMICAL APPEARANCE, SKIN INDENTATION AND LOCAL NERVE DAMAGE (numbness or loss of muscle function).**

**I (we)** understand that anesthesia involves additional risks and hazards but **I (we)** request the use of anesthetics for the relief and protection from pain during the planned and additional procedures.

**I (we)** have been given an opportunity to ask questions of my physicians about my condition, alternative forms of anesthesia and treatment, risks of non-treatment, the procedures to use, and the risks and hazards involved, and **I (we)** believe that **I (we)** have sufficient information to give this informed consent.

**I (we)** certify this form has been fully explained to me, that **I (we)** have read it or have had it read to me, that the blank spaces have been filled in, and that **I (we)** understand its contents.

**PATIENT Signature:** _____

**Or other Legally Responsible Person Signature:** _____/

**Relationship:** _____

**Date:** _____

**Witness:** _____ **Date:** _____

**I have explained to the patient or legal representative the disclosure and consent required for the medical, surgical, and/ or diagnostic procedures planned as well as the patient's right to withhold consent.**

**Physician's Signature:** _____ **Date:** _____

transient, a throbbing sensation after freezing the digits may persist for 1–2 hours. An individual who has previously experienced debilitating pain after cryosurgery is likely to want a local anesthetic if further treatment is needed. Most importantly, patients should be offered the option for a local anesthetic if the planned treatment is likely to cause significant and prolonged pain.

In general, short single-freeze schedules used for benign or premalignant skin lesions will not require local anesthesia. Topical agents such as tetracaine and a eutectic mixture of lidocaine and prilocaine (EMLA) may be applied 30–60 min before a procedure for the treatment of warts in children. The most effective form of local anesthesia is by injection of lidocaine with or without epinephrine. We prefer to use lidocaine with epinephrine (unless there is a contraindication to epinephrine use) because there is a smaller risk of lidocaine toxicity and the anesthesia will last longer. This will make the treatment itself painless but also provide pain relief for a few hours after the procedure. The decision to use this approach must be determined by

the patient's wishes. Injectable lidocaine is the preferred method of anesthesia used before treating skin cancers with cryosurgery. More prolonged pain should be managed with analgesic tablets such as acetaminophen or ibuprofen.

## MONITORING OF TEMPERATURE

Some of the original cryosurgery research used thermocouples (temperature-measuring devices that can withstand extreme cold and hot temperatures) and pigskin to study ice-ball formation. The aim was to look at the relationship between diameter and depth of freeze and between duration of freeze (using the spot-freeze method) and temperature at various depths. The results were translated into guidelines for the use of the spot-freeze technique in the treatment of basal cell carcinoma. During routine practice in the treatment of benign lesions and superficial skin cancers, monitoring is not required.

The Cry-Ac TrackerCam is a new device that measures the temperature of the skin when spraying liquid nitrogen using the infrared sensor technology. The infrared sensors

*Box 6.2* Declaración y Consentimiento Criocirugía

**PARA EL PACIENTE: Usted, como paciente, tiene derecho a ser informado sobre su condición y sobre los recomendados procedimientos de criocirugía que serán utilizados para que así usted tome la decisión de aceptar realizarse el procedimiento o no, una vez que sepa los riesgos y peligros involucrados. Hay muchos beneficios a la criocirugía, incluyendo la erradicación de la enfermedad de la piel a tratar. Esta declaración no tiene la intención de asustarlo o alarmarlo, es simplemente un esfuerzo para que usted esté mejor informado para poder dar o negar su consentimiento para el procedimiento.**

Yo (**nosotros**) solicito (amos) de manera voluntaria que el Dr. _____

como mi médico, junto con sus socios, ayudantes técnicos y otros proveedores médicos que consideren necesarios, me proporcionen el tratamiento para mi condición, el cual se me ha explicado como.

Yo (**nosotros**) voluntariamente acepto y autorizo criocirugía con _____

Así como pueden existir riesgos y peligros en seguir con mi condiciónes actual sin tratamiento, también existen riesgos y peligros relacionados con la realización de criocirugía. Yo (**nosotros**) también entiendo (entendemos) que pueden presentarse los siguientes riesgos y peligros en conexión con este procedimiento en particular:

**DOLOR, HINCHAZON, AMPOLLAS, CAMBIO DE PIGMENTACIóN EN EL AREA DE TRATAMIENTO, CURACIóN LENTA, SANGRADO, INFECCIóN, CICATRI-CES, NUEVO CRECIMIENTO, CAMBIO EN LA APARIEN-CIA ANATóMICA, HENDIDURA EN LA PIEL Y DAñO A LOS NERVIOS LOCALES (sensación de entumecimiento o pérdida de la función muscular).**

Yo (**nosotros**) entiendo (entendemos) que la anestesia involucra riesgos y peligros adicionales, pero **yo** (**nosotros**) solicito (solicitamos) el uso de anestésicos para el alivio y la protección contra el dolor durante los procedimientos previstos y los adicionales.

Se me (nos) ha ofrecido la oportunidad de hacer preguntas sobre mi padecimiento., las formas alternativas de anestesia y tratamiento, los riesgos por no recibir tratamiento, los procedimientos que se utilizarán y los riesgos y peligros involucrados, y creo (creemos) que tengo (tenemos) la información suficiente para dar este consentimiento informado.

Yo (**nosotros**) certifico (certificamos) que este formulario se me (nos) ha sido plenamente explicado., que **yo** (**nosotros**) lo he leído o se me ha leído, que los espacios en blanco han sido llenados y que **yo** (**nosotros**) entiendo (entendemos) su contenido.

FIRMA DEL PACIENTE: _____

O de otra persona legalmente responsable: _____

Parentesco: _____

Fecha: _____

Testigo: _____

Fecha: _____

**Le he explicado al paciente o su representante legal la divulgación y consentimiento necesarios para la realización de los procedimientos médicos, quirúrgicos y / o diagnósticos programados, así como el derecho del paciente a rehusar su consentimiento.**

Firma del Médico: _____ Fecha: _____

---

*Box 6.3* Aftercare Instructions: What to Expect After Cryosurgery

Your skin lesion has been treated with liquid nitrogen (or another refrigerant). The tissue was destroyed by freezing it to a low temperature. You may have discomfort, burning, or pain after the treatment. Your skin may become red and swollen, and weep fluid, or a blister may form. A small blister should be covered with an adhesive dressing. If a large blister develops, let out the fluid with a sterile pointed instrument, repeat if the blister refills, and apply a sterile dressing until it stops draining.

Wound infections are uncommon but sometimes the surface may look yellow. If you suspect a wound infection please contact your doctor. Dressings that can absorb fluid may be used to prevent the wound sticking to garments. Treatments on the face and scalp may lead to a headache after the procedure. The lesion, or part of it, may peel or drop off in a week or two and a further scaly crust may form on the wound.

Sometimes the smallest nerve endings in the skin can be damaged so that the treated area feels numb. Cryosurgery may leave the treated area a little lighter or darker.

If the lesion fails to respond completely or if it reforms you may require further treatment. If you have any cause for concern please contact your doctor for advice.

---

*Box 6.4* Cryosurgery Procedure Note

**Procedure: cryosurgery**

Using liquid nitrogen with: cryospray, cryoprobe or forceps.

**Locations:**

**Number of lesions treated:**

Patient was advised of the nature and purpose of the cryosurgery, alternate therapies, risks, and complications (pain, swelling, blisters, change in pigmentation in the treated area, slow healing, bleeding, infection, scarring, regrowth, change in anatomic appearance, skin indentation, and local nerve damage).

Informed consent obtained.

Lesions were treated with cryosurgery.

There were no immediate complications.

Advised on wound care.

Follow-up instructions provided.

---

were calibrated using thermocouples. All clinicians do not need this more expensive top-of-the-line cryogun for the practice of cryosurgery. It is very helpful in building confidence for the treatment of skin cancers with cryosurgery because it is the only unit that provides feedback on the temperatures achieved (see Chapter 3 for additional information).

## RECORD KEEPING

For legal, audit, and research purposes accurate records should be kept for each cryosurgical procedure carried out. Information to consider includes the following:[1]

- Effects of previous treatments (if any)
- Lesions treated
- Technique used
- Tip type or aperture
- Number of freeze–thaw cycles
- Length of freeze time if measured
- Halo diameter around lesion
- Patient tolerability
- Adverse events
- Aftercare instructions/adjunct therapies.

This information could be stored in individual patient records. Clinicians with modern software packages for practice management may be able to bring together all their cryosurgical treatments for analysis. Those without such packages, but who would like to audit their practice, would need to keep a database in addition to the individual records (see sample procedure note in Box 6.4).

## FOLLOW-UP

Patients undergoing cryosurgery should have follow-up appropriate for the lesion and its treatment. There are several reasons that follow-up may be required either soon after the treatment or in the longer term:

- Wound check
- Management of side effects/complications
- Repeat treatment for same or other lesions
- Possibility of persistent or recurrent tumor
- Examination to detect skin cancers on sun-damaged skin.

Even when armed with good wound-care information some patients are frightened by the site of their cryosurgical wound with swelling or blistering, and telephone for an urgent evaluation. If the first phase of healing progresses satisfactorily it is still instructive and helpful to doctor and patient alike to check the cryosurgery site some time from 4 weeks to 12 weeks after treatment (except in instances when small benign lesions have been treated and have resolved). This provides a useful opportunity to assess the clinical and cosmetic outcome of treatment. Some conditions such as warts and keloids will require further treatment, whereas individuals with multiple seborrheic or actinic keratoses may wish to have additional lesions treated.

Follow-up after skin cancer treatment is important. In the short term the finding of tumor at the site of cryotherapy should be regarded as persistent rather than recurrent disease. In a paper by Rowe et al., the authors reviewed all papers on recurrence rates after treatment of primary basal cell carcinoma with any modality.[2] They found that less than a third of all recurrences appear in the first year after treatment, only 50% appear within the first 2 years after treatment, and only 66% appear within the first 3 years after treatment. The 5-year recurrence rate after cryotherapy was 7.5%.[2] We suggest initial follow-up after skin cancer treatment at 3–6 months and every 6–12 months after that. Of course this schedule needs to take into account the types and locations of skin cancers treated, the patient risk factors for new skin cancers, and the patient resources for accessing medical care.

## REFERENCES

1. Perfect H, Price AM, Reeken S, Ryan S, Stephen K, Woodward C. Best practice in cryosurgery. A statement for health care professionals. Dermatol Nursing 2012;10(2 suppl).
2. Rowe DE, Carroll RJ, Day CL. Long-term recurrence rates in previously untreated (primary) basal cell carcinoma: implications for patient follow-up. J Dermatol Surg Oncol 1989;15:315–28.

The number of published studies of cryosurgery in dermatology is small in comparison to other areas of medicine. At the end of 2013 a US National Library of Medicine (PubMed) search on the terms "cryosurgery" or "cryotherapy" and "dermatology" yielded only 822 results and only 102 of these were clinical trials. On the same day a search of "psoriasis" yielded over 34 000 results with over 2700 clinical trials. Of course topics such as hypertension yield over 300 000 results with close to 30 000 clinical trials. That said, the purpose of this chapter is not to review all 100 clinical trials but to focus on the best existing evidence for three common cryosurgery indications: warts, actinic keratoses, and basal cell carcinoma. We have chosen three examples from the spectrum of benign to premalignant to malignant lesions, which are the best studied lesions representing the spectrum.

## WARTS

All studies of cryosurgery of warts are limited in their quality. Four of the largest and best studies were chosen for analysis.

### Berth-Jones J, Hutchinson PE. Modern treatment of warts: cure rates at 3 and 6 months. Br J Dermatol 1992;127:262–5.

#### Study Description

Four hundred consecutive referrals with viral warts of the hands and/or feet were investigated to determine the cure rate from a combination of cryotherapy, keratolytic wart paint, and paring. For treatment failures after 3 months, the value of continuing cryotherapy and additional treatment with the immunomodulator inosine pranobex was assessed. Participants were treated for 3 months with wart paint and cryotherapy, and were randomized to receive, or not, paring in addition. Those who did not respond by 3 months were randomized to receive, or not, 3 months of further cryotherapy, and to receive inosine pranobex 60 mg/kg per day for 1 week each month, or matching placebo. Of the participants, 52% were cured by 3 months. The chance of cure was inversely related to both the length of history and the diameter of the largest wart. Paring improved the cure rate for plantar warts but not for hand warts. During the second 3 months the cure rate fell to 41%. Neither cryotherapy nor inosine pranobex significantly improved this response.

#### Comments

This study attempts to investigate cure rates of cryosurgery of common warts in combination with other therapies. Even when combining cryosurgery with keratolytic wart painting and paring only 52% of participants were cured by 3 months. Larger warts and warts with longer duration are more difficult to cure.

### Ahmed I, Agarwal S, Ilchyshyn A, Charles-Holmes S, Berth-Jones J. Liquid nitrogen cryotherapy of common warts: cryo-spray vs. cotton wool bud. Br J Dermatol 2001;144:1006–9.

This prospective study of 207 patients was undertaken to compare cryospray versus cotton wool bud with regard to cure rate after 3 months of treatment.

**Methods**: Patients referred to two hospital dermatology departments with hand or foot warts were allocated to have liquid nitrogen applied with either a cryospray or a cotton-wool bud. Using either technique, liquid nitrogen was applied until ice-ball formation had spread from the center to include a margin of 2 mm around each wart. Treatment was done every 2 weeks for up to 3 months. Plantar warts were pared and treated with a double freeze–thaw cycle. The endpoint of the study was complete clearance of all warts.

**Results**: 363 patients were enrolled, mean age 21 years (range 3–75), 188 male and 175 female. The mean duration of the warts was 98 weeks (median 78, range 2–936). The number of warts on the hands and feet varied from 1 to 80 (mean 5). The treatment groups were comparable with regard to baseline demographics; 207 patients were evaluable. Cure rates at 3 months were 47% in the cotton-wool bud group and 44% in the cryospray group ($p = 0.8$). Warts that had been present for 6 months or less ($n = 31$) had a greater chance of clearance (84%) compared with warts that had been present for more than 6 months (39%, $n = 176$) ($p < 0.0005$).

**Conclusions**: Cryotherapy with liquid nitrogen for hand and foot warts in this study was equally effective when applied with a cotton-wool bud or by means of a spray.

#### Comments

Cryospray is capable of producing lower freeze temperatures than liquid nitrogen applied with a cotton-wool bud. However, in this relatively large prospective study the cryospray technique did not produce higher cure rates than the cotton-wool bud method. The authors froze the hand and foot warts until a 2-mm halo margin had been obtained with the ice-ball formation. Therefore freeze times were not used or recorded. Only the plantar warts were pared and received a double freeze–thaw cycle. The cure rates at 3 months were 47% in the cotton-wool bud group and 44% in the cryospray group – not very impressive overall. The cure rates may have been higher if a double freeze–thaw cycle had been used on the hand warts as well. As in the previous study, warts of shorter duration are more likely to be cured.

**Connolly M, Bazmi K, O'Connell M, Lyons JF, Bourke JF. Cryotherapy of viral warts: a sustained 10-s freeze is more effective than the traditional method. Br J Dermatol 2001;145:554–7.**

Two hundred patients enrolled.

**Objectives**: To compare the efficacy of the traditional freeze (halo of ice around the wart) and a more aggressive sustained 10-s freeze in the treatment of common viral warts with liquid nitrogen.

**Methods**: Patients attending a dedicated wart clinic were randomized to receive either a traditional freeze or a 10-s sustained freeze with liquid nitrogen delivered by a spray gun. Of the 200 patients recruited, 100 were in each group.

**Results**: After 5 treatments, 49 patients in the 10-s freeze group were clear of warts (64% of non-defaulters) compared with 31 (39%) of those in the traditional freeze group ($\chi^2 = 6.7$; $p = 0.009$). Seventy-four patients in the 10-s freeze group, compared with 59 in the traditional freeze group, had either improved or cleared after five treatments ($\chi^2 = 5.0$; $p = 0.02$). Morbidity was significantly greater in the 10-s freeze group; 64 patients suffered pain or blistering compared with 44 in the traditional freeze group ($\chi^2 = 10.8$; $p = 0.0045$). Five patients were withdrawn from the 10-s freeze group because of pain compared with one patient in the traditional freeze group.

**Conclusions**: A 10-s sustained freeze is more effective in the cryotherapy of viral warts but carries a significantly greater morbidity in terms of pain and blistering.

**Comments**

This study compared the technique of freezing until a halo of ice around wart is achieved versus sustaining the ice ball for a further 10 seconds. The longer freeze time was more effective in this study but was more painful and produced more blistering than the halo freeze group. This is important and reminds us that information given to the patient about side effects must reflect the extent of cryosurgery. It also helps to keep in perspective the likely side effects that might be expected if one were to follow recommendations for 20- to 30-second freeze times without anesthesia.

We prefer to use shorter freeze times using halo diameter as a guide, but using a double freeze–thaw cycle.

**Khaled A, Ben RS, Kharfi M, Zeglaoui F, Fazaa B, Kamoun MR. Assessment of cryotherapy by liquid nitrogen in the treatment of hand and feet warts. Tunis Med 2009;87:690–2.**

The aim of this study of 100 patients was to determine factors influencing therapeutic response of warts to cryotherapy by liquid nitrogen.

**Methods**: It was a prospective transversal study including 100 patients with warts of the hands and/or feet treated with the cotton-wool bud method. Patients received one treatment/week with a maximum of four sessions. Patients whose warts were seen to be resolved were classified as cured. Cure-predictive factors were studied with a multi-varied analysis using logistic regression.

**Results**: Of the 100 patients (56 females/44 males, mean age: 22 years), 10 were withdrawn. In 89 patients, warts were present on the hands, whereas 23 had warts on the feet and 12 on both the hands and the feet. The mean number of warts per patient was seven. The total cure rate was of 64.4% and was higher in hands compared with feet (70.8% vs. 10.5%). There was no difference between the mean ages of those who were cured or not cured (22.2 years vs. 21 years). The mean duration of warts in cured patients was lower than that for patients who were not cured. The mean number of warts before treatment was 4.3 in cured patients and 12.3 warts in not cured patients. The mean number of treatments was 2.3 in cured patients and 4 in not cured patients.

**Conclusion**: The effectiveness of liquid nitrogen in the treatment of hand and feet warts seems to depend on multiple factors: the wart's duration, the number of warts, and the number of treatments.

**Comments**

Although this study was performed solely using the cotton-wool bud we can still generalize some of the effectiveness factors to all forms of liquid nitrogen application. This study confirmed the findings of other studies that longstanding warts and multiple warts are more difficult to cure. Early responders tended to have a better outcome.

**ACTINIC KERATOSES**

All studies of cryosurgery of actinic keratoses are limited in their quality and some of the comparative studies are manufacturer sponsored. Four of the largest and best studies were chosen for analysis.

**Thai KE, Fergin P, Freeman M, et al. A prospective study of the use of cryosurgery for the treatment of actinic keratoses. Int J Dermatol 2004;43:687–92.**

The aim of this study was to determine prospectively the true efficacy of cryosurgery as a treatment for actinic keratoses in everyday dermatologic practice.

**Methods**: A prospective, multicentered study (a subsidiary study of a photodynamic therapy trial) was performed. Patients with untreated actinic keratoses >5 mm in diameter on the face and scalp were recruited. Eligible lesions received a single freeze–thaw cycle with liquid nitrogen given via a spray device and were reviewed 3 months thereafter. Each center used their preferred freeze time. The freeze time was measured as the time from the formation of an ice ball to the start of thawing. The only treatment criterion was complete freezing of actinic keratoses and a 1-mm rim of normal skin. Treated lesions were assessed as complete or non-complete response.

**Results**: Ninety adults from the community with 421 eligible actinic keratoses were recruited. The overall individual complete response rate was 67.2% (standard error of the mean [SEM] = ±3.5%; 95% confidence interval [CI] = 60.4–74.1%). Complete response was 39% for freeze times of <5 s, 69% for freeze times >5 s, and 83% for freeze times >20 s. Cosmetic outcomes were good to excellent in 94% of complete response lesions. The main adverse events were pain, stinging, and burning during treatment, and hypopigmentation after healing.

**Conclusions**: Cryosurgery is an effective treatment for actinic keratoses. The true complete response rate is significantly lower than that previously reported. The freeze duration influences successful treatment. Adverse events are mild and well tolerated.

## Comments

This is the best study of cryosurgery for actinic keratoses published (Table 7.1). It is not manufacturer sponsored and the quality of the study design is excellent. The results should be applied to determine appropriate freeze times in clinical practice. Although the study dealt only with actinic keratoses of the face and scalp, the data can also be used to guide treatment for lesions of the extremities and trunk. Although the actinic keratoses were >5 mm in diameter there are no data about their thickness. In general, thicker lesions need longer freeze times. However, we see that <5 seconds of freeze time had a low cure rate of 39% and of >5 seconds increased the cure rate to 69%. Although

over 20 seconds of freeze time had a higher cure rate of 83%, the patients reported increased pain. From the wart study above, freeze times >10 seconds are noted to have greater pain and blistering. Double freeze–thaw cycles were not used, so we know the results only of a single freeze time. When patients are finding a prolonged freeze to be painful the freeze time can be split into two freeze–thaw cycles.

**Morton C, Campbell S, Gupta G, et al. Intraindividual, right-left comparison of topical methyl aminolaevulinate-photodynamic therapy and cryotherapy in subjects with actinic keratoses: a multicentre, randomized controlled study. Br J Dermatol 2006;155:1029–36.**

The primary objective was to compare the lesion response and patient preference for topical methyl aminolevulinate (MAL)–photodynamic therapy (PDT) versus cryotherapy for the treatment of actinic keratosis of the face and scalp.

**Methods**: In this 24-week, multicenter, randomized, intraindividual (right–left) study, participants received both one treatment session of MAL–PDT and a double freeze–thaw cryotherapy; the treatments were randomly allocated to either side of the face/scalp. Double freeze–thaw cryotherapy was performed using liquid nitrogen spray, with an applicator size selected to achieve a 1- to 2-mm frozen rim outside the marked outline of the lesion. Lesions with a non-complete response were retreated after 12 weeks. The primary assessments were the participant's overall preference and lesion response at week 24. Secondary assessments included lesion response at week 12, cosmetic outcome, participant and investigator cosmetic outcome preference at week 24, and investigator overall preference at week 24. Skin discomfort and adverse events were also evaluated.

**Results**: In total, 119 participants with 1501 lesions were included in the study. At week 12, treatment with MAL–PDT resulted in a significantly higher rate of cured lesions relative to cryotherapy (percentage lesion reduction from baseline: 86.9% vs. 76.2%; $p <0.001$). At week 24, both treatment groups showed a high rate of cured lesions (89.1% for MAL–PDT vs. 86.1% for cryotherapy; $p = 0.20$; 95% CI: −1.62 to 7.67). Results for participant and investigator preferences, as well as cosmetic outcome, favored MAL–PDT. Both treatment regimens were safe and well tolerated.

**Conclusions**: The present study shows that, when treated with both MAL–PDT and cryotherapy, participants significantly prefer MAL–PDT treatment for actinic keratoses. MAL–PDT is an attractive treatment option for actinic keratoses, with comparable efficacy and superior cosmetic outcomes compared with double freeze–thaw cryotherapy.

*Table 7.1* Actinic Keratoses of the Face and Scalp >5 mm – Cure Rates with a **Single** Freeze

| Single freeze time (s) | Cure rate (%) |
| --- | --- |
| <5 | 39 |
| 5–20 | 69 |
| >20 | 83 |

**Conflicts of interest**: Seven of the authors received funding from Galderma as investigators of this study, and three were employees of Galderma. Other declared conflicts of interest were with Galderma and 3M Healthcare.

## Comments

This study gives us the benefit of data based on the double freeze–thaw technique. In addition halo diameters of 1–2 mm were achieved. The 6-month cure rates of 86.1% for cryotherapy are excellent and statistically equal to the cure rates using PDT. The paper emphasizes that participants and investigators preferred the cosmetic outcome of PDT but we need to recognize a strong manufacturer influence on the study and writing of the results. Despite this bias, the data for cryotherapy are helpful.

**Kaufmann R, Spelman L, Weightman W, et al. Multicentre intraindividual randomized trial of topical methyl aminolaevulinate-photodynamic therapy vs cryotherapy for multiple actinic keratoses on the extremities. Br J Dermatol 2008;158:994–9.**

The aims of this study were to compare efficacy, safety, cosmetic outcome, and patient preference of methyl aminolevulinate–photodynamic therapy (MAL–PDT) versus cryotherapy in patients with non-face/scalp actinic keratoses.

**Methods**: A multicenter, controlled, randomized, open, intraindividual, right–left comparison was performed. Patients with non-hyperkeratotic actinic keratosis were treated once with MAL–PDT and cryotherapy on either side of the body. Double freeze–thaw cryosurgery was performed using a liquid nitrogen spray, with an applicator size selected to achieve a 1- to 2-mm frozen rim outside the marked outline of the actinic keratosis. The timing of the freeze–thaw application was performed according to the usual practice of each investigating center. At week 12, lesions showing non-complete response were retreated. The primary efficacy variable was the lesion response at week 24. Investigator's assessment of cosmetic outcome, patient's preference in terms of cosmetic outcome, and a patient preference questionnaire were also analyzed at week 24.

**Results**: In total, of 121 patients with 1343 lesions (98% located on the extremities and the remainder on the trunk and neck) were included. Both treatments provided a high mean percentage reduction in lesion count at week 24, with significantly higher efficacy for cryotherapy: 78% for MAL–PDT and 88% for cryotherapy ($p = 0.002$, per protocol population). Investigator's assessment of cosmetic outcome was significantly better for MAL–PDT than cryotherapy ($p < 0.001$), 79% of lesions having an excellent cosmetic outcome with MAL–PDT vs. 56% with cryotherapy at week 24. The cosmetic outcome achieved by MAL–PDT compared with cryotherapy was also preferred by patients (50% vs. 22%, respectively, $p < 0.001$), and 59% of patients would prefer to have any new lesions treated with MAL–PDT compared with 25% with cryotherapy ($p < 0.001$). Both treatment regimens were safe and well tolerated.

**Conclusions**: MAL–PDT showed inferior efficacy for treatment of non-face/scalp actinic keratosis compared with cryotherapy. However, both treatments showed high efficacy, and MAL–PDT conveyed the advantages of better cosmesis and higher patient preference.

**Conflicts of interest**: This study was funded by Galderma. Seven of the authors received funding support from Galderma to conduct this study, and three were employees of Galderma.

## Comments

This study is very similar to the preceding one with a strong manufacturer influence. In this case the cryotherapy efficacy of 88% at 6 months was significantly higher than the PDT result of 78%. The investigators did report greater patient preference for the PDT. Similar to the preceding study the methodology used involved a double freeze–thaw cycle with a 1- to 2-mm halo diameter.

**Krawtchenko N, Roewert-Huber J, Ulrich M, Mann I, Sterry W, Stockfleth E. A randomised study of topical 5% imiquimod vs. topical 5-fluorouracil vs cryosurgery in immunocompetent patients with actinic keratoses: a comparison of clinical and histological outcomes including 1-year follow-up. Br J Dermatol 2007;157(suppl 2):34–40.**

This study compared the initial and 12-month clinical clearance, histologic clearance, and cosmetic outcomes of topically applied 5% imiquimod cream, 5% 5-fluorouracil (5-FU) ointment, and cryosurgery for the treatment of actinic keratoses. **Patients/Methods**: Patients were randomized to one of the following three treatment groups: one or two courses of cryosurgery (20–40 s of cryospray per lesion), topical 5-FU (twice daily for 4 weeks), or one or two courses of topical imiquimod (three times per week for 4 weeks each).

**Results**: Sixty-eight percent (17/25) of patients treated with cryosurgery, 96% (23/24) of patients treated with 5-FU, and 85% (22/26) of patients treated with imiquimod achieved initial clinical clearance ($p = 0.03$). The histologic clearance rate for cryosurgery was 32% (8/25), 67% (16/24) for 5-FU, and 73% (19/26) in the imiquimod group ($p = 0.03$). The 12-month follow-up showed a high rate of recurrent and new lesions in the 5-FU and cryosurgery arms. The sustained clearance rate of initially cleared individual lesions was 28% (7/25) for cryosurgery, 54% (13/24) for 5-FU, and 73% (19/26) for imiquimod ($p < 0.01$). Sustained clearance of the total treatment field was 4% (1/25), 33% (8/24), and 73% (19/26) of patients after cryosurgery, 5-FU, and imiquimod, respectively ($p < 0.01$). The patients in the IMIQ group were judged to have the best cosmetic outcomes ($p = 0.0001$).

**Conclusion:** Imiquimod treatment of actinic keratoses resulted in superior sustained clearance and cosmetic outcomes compared with cryosurgery and 5-FU. It should be considered as a first-line therapy for sustained treatment of actinic keratoses.

Note that ES acts as a consultant to Meda Pharma, the company that manufactures 5% imiquimod.

### Comments

This is an unusual study in that the cryosurgery was more aggressive than the other studies and the outcomes are far less effective. The investigators used 20–40 seconds of cryospray freeze time without anesthesia. We rarely freeze over 20–30 seconds without lidocaine anesthesia for benign or premalignant lesions. This is the only study that performed biopsies to determine clearance rates. The data presented here shows imiquimod to be far superior to 5-FU and cryosurgery, but it is such an outlier that it is hard to know what to make of this study. One author is a consultant for the manufacturer of imiquimod but did not declare this as a conflict of interest. This is concerning. It is clear that imiquimod and 5-FU are standard treatments for actinic keratoses, especially when field therapy is desired.

We would not drop the use of cryosurgery as the first line of treatment for individual actinic keratoses from the evidence in this study. Nor would we use a 20- to 40-second freeze time for actinic keratoses. The data from the first three studies should best guide cryosurgery of actinic keratoses with a minimum of 5 s freeze time, 1–2 mm of halo diameter, and a strong consideration for a double freeze–thaw cycle (especially for thicker actinic keratoses). In general, thicker actinic keratoses should be treated more aggressively than the thinner ones. If an actinic keratosis is so large and thick that it needs a 30-s freeze time it may be prudent to take a biopsy to rule out Bowen's disease. Freeze times of 20–40 s or more are best performed with local anesthetic (injectable lidocaine as the gold standard).

### BASAL CELL CARCINOMA
**Mallon E, Dawber R. Cryosurgery in the treatment of basal cell carcinoma. Assessment of one and two freeze-thaw cycle schedules. Dermatol Surg 1996;22:854–8.**

This study compared the efficacy of one freeze–thaw cycle versus two freeze-thaw cycles in the treatment of facial basal cell carcinomas (BCCs). In addition, it investigated the efficacy of one freeze–thaw cycle in the treatment of superficial truncal BCCs. This was investigated in a prospective, randomized, post-treatment, follow-up study. Eight-four facial BCCs were treated with either a single 30-s freeze–thaw cycle or a double 30-second freeze–thaw

cycle (randomly assigned). Second, 29 superficial truncal BCCs were treated with a single 30-s freeze–thaw cycle. A 95.3% cure rate was achieved in the treatment of facial BCCs with a double freeze–thaw cycle. This compared with a cure rate of only 79.4% when facial lesions were treated with a single freeze–thaw cycle. Treatment of superficial truncal BCCs with a single freeze–thaw cycle achieved a cure rate of 95.5%.

### Comments

Facial BCCs should receive a double 30-s freeze–thaw cycle with liquid nitrogen. One 30-s freeze–thaw cycle to superficial truncal BCCs appears adequate. Note that nodular truncal BCCs were not studied so that it might be best to use a 30-s freeze–thaw cycle for these thicker tumors. Local anesthesia is suggested for such long freeze times.

**Peikert JM. Prospective trial of curettage and cryosurgery in the management of non-facial, superficial, and minimally invasive basal and squamous cell carcinoma. Int J Dermatol 2011;50:1135–8.**

This study seeks to determine the long-term cure rate associated with curettage and cryosurgery in the treatment of small, non-facial, superficial basal and squamous cell carcinomas. 69 patients with 100 non-facial tumors, ≤2 cm in diameter, consisting of superficial basal cell carcinoma (BCC), superficial nodular BCC with papillary dermal invasion, squamous cell carcinoma (SCC) *in situ*, and SCC with papillary dermal invasion were prospectively treated with curettage and cryotherapy, and subsequently evaluated at 1- and 5-year intervals. No tumor recurred after 1 year of follow-up, and one recurrence occurred within the 5-year interval, for a 99% recurrence-free endpoint.

**Details of treatment method:** 4-mm margins were drawn around the visible border of each tumor. Local anesthesia was then placed using 1% lidocaine with 1:100 000 parts epinephrine. Curettage was then performed in multiple directions with a sharp, disposable 2-mm curette until all friable tumor tissue and epidermis had been removed from within the marked margins, leaving a clinically uniform, normal-appearing, normal-feeling dermal base. Hemostasis was achieved with 20% aluminum chloride. The entire curetted field was then treated broadly using a continuous liquid nitrogen spray, aimed at a distance of 5 mm, using a paint brush method, for one freeze–thaw cycle with freeze times of 10–20 s, with variation based on the size of the field being treated.

### Comments

This study supports the authors' conclusion that curettage and cryosurgery are a highly effective and reliable treatment method for select, low-risk, non-melanoma skin cancers off the face and ≤2 cm in diameter. Note that aluminum chloride was used for hemostasis rather than Monsel's solution. Also, a single freeze–thaw cycle was used with relatively short freeze times of 10–20 s. This should be compared with the Mallon paper above in which their single freeze–thaw cycle (for lesions on the trunk) was 30 s. However, the curettage does debulk the tumor so that it is reasonable to believe that a shorter freeze time may be effective.

### Jaramillo-Ayerbe F. Cryosurgery in difficult to treat basal cell carcinoma. Int J Dermatol 2000;39:223–9.

The purpose of the study was to establish the cure rate, functional preservation, cosmetic results, acceptance, and complications of cryosurgery in difficult-to-treat BCCs; 136 consecutive patients with 171 difficult-to-treat BCCs (because of size >1 cm, location, nature, or patient condition) were treated by the **mixed technique of curettage followed by liquid nitrogen application**. After an average follow-up of 5.2 years (6 months to 9.1 years), a cure rate of 91.8% was achieved. The treatment was well tolerated, widely accepted by the patients, of low cost, and with good functional and cosmetic results. The authors concluded that curettage and cryosurgery offer an acceptable cure rate with good functional and cosmetic results in difficult-to-treat BCCs.

### Comments
Curettage and cryosurgery combined may be considered as a treatment option even in patients with difficult-to-treat BCCs. All patients received local anesthesia with lidocaine and epinephrine. Lesions were curetted with small diameter curettes (2–4 mm) and Monsel's solution was applied to achieve hemostasis. Liquid nitrogen was delivered by spray technique or cryoprobes and a double freeze–thaw cycle was used. The ocular globe was protected with a Jaeger lid plate or a corneal shield on palpebrally located lesions. There were some significant complications such as nasal cartilage necrosis that needed surgical reconstruction and four patients had wound infections requiring oral antibiotics. Many of the eyelids treated developed ectropion which partially resolved after several months. The cosmetic results were considered unfavorable on the lips. Although the use of cryosurgery was employed for these difficult-to-treat BCCs, Mohs' micrographic surgery, when available, would likely be the treatment of choice for tumors around the eyelids, lips, and nose. The study is included to show the opportunities that cryosurgery can provide rather than to recommend cryosurgery over Mohs' surgery for difficult-to-treat BCCs.

### Kokoszka A, Scheinfeld N. Evidence-based review of the use of cryosurgery in treatment of basal cell carcinoma. Dermatol Surg 2003;29:566–71.

This systematic review found 13 non-controlled prospective studies and 4 randomized clinical trials comparing cryosurgery with other methods of treatment for BCCs. Recurrence rates of BCCs treated with cryosurgery are low (<10%). Except in one study, recurrence rates are calculated based on clinical, rather than histologic, diagnosis. Cosmetic results of cryosurgery treatment are described as good by most investigators. Overall, there are sufficient data to consider cryosurgery as a reasonable treatment for BCCs. There are no good studies comparing cryosurgery with other modalities. Also, there is no evidence on whether curetting the lesions before cryosurgery affects the efficacy of treatment.

### Comments
This is the best systematic review of the use of cryosurgery for BCCs. Recurrence rates of less than 10% are comparable to surgical excision and electrodessication and curettage. Although there is no evidence that curetting the lesions before cryosurgery affects the efficacy of treatment, there is good evidence that this is a reasonable treatment methodology based on two studies cited above. However, curettage before cryosurgery is a choice not currently supported by comparison studies.

### Thissen MR, Nieman FH, Ideler AH, et al. Cosmetic results of cryosurgery versus surgical excision for primary uncomplicated basal cell carcinomas of the head and neck. Dermatol Surg 2000;26:759–64.

Cosmetic results after cryosurgery and excision (prospective randomized study) of primary BCCs in the head/neck area were assessed by five professional observers and the patients; 96 BCCs were treated either with surgical excision ($n = 48$) or cryosurgery ($n = 48$). Clinical professionals evaluated the cosmetic results after surgery as significantly better. The beautician had no preference for either therapy. The patients had a significant preference for excision. Localization and size of the tumor did not modify this general preference for excision.

**Cryosurgery methodology**: Thorough curettage using a sharp curette was performed under local anesthesia (lidocaine 1% without epinephrine). Initially a large curette (no. 3) was used to debulk the tumor mass. Finally, a small curette (no. 1) was used to remove the remainder of the BCC around the borders. Monsel's solution was used to perform hemostasis. A liquid nitrogen spray was used to freeze the tissue. Freezing was carried out in two freezing periods, each lasting 20 s. The halo thaw time between these cycles was 60 s. All tumors were treated with the cone-spray technique, using a neoprene cone with a wall thickness of 2 mm. The cone was modeled to the proper shape to enclose the tumor and a free margin of 5 mm around the tumor, and was pressed firmly against the underlying (bony) structure. If the tumor was too wide to be enclosed by the cone, freezing was performed in sections.

## Comments

Cryosurgery generally leaves a round hypopigmented scar and surgical excision should leave a linear scar unless a flap or graft is required. It is not surprising that the surgical scar was often preferred cosmetically over the cryosurgery scar in appearance. It is interesting that the beautician had no preference for the cosmetic result of one method over the other, possibly because the longer linear scar may also have railroad track marks, and this pattern is not better in appearance to a shorter round scar. Cosmetic concerns are only one factor involved in the decision of which therapy will be employed for the treatment of BCC. Given the many other factors involved, cryosurgery is a reasonable treatment option for many patients with the diagnosis of BCC.

## CONCLUSION

Despite the relatively small number of studies on cryosurgery, an evidence-based approach is used in the chapters that follow. Chapters 8–10 deal with cryosurgery of benign, premalignant, and malignant conditions, respectively, and utilize available evidence to inform practice recommendations.

# 8    Benign lesions

This chapter deals with the management of benign lesions and therefore constitutes a major part of cryosurgical practice. Most benign lesions are treated for cosmetic reasons and there is a balance to be achieved between the simplicity and effectiveness of the treatment, on the one hand, and the discomfort and side effects, on the other. Some lesions, especially those arising in the epidermis, respond predictably and cryosurgery may be the most effective or least invasive option. Other lesions (eg keloids) respond unpredictably and cryosurgery is only one of many modalities that should be discussed with the patient.

## HOW EFFECTIVE IS CRYOSURGERY?
Cryosurgery is generally regarded as one of the mainstays of treatment for viral warts and seborrheic keratoses. The cure rates are moderately good for viral warts with a success rate of 54% with "aggressive cryosurgery."[1] It is wise to be cautiously optimistic because sometimes even innocuous-looking warts can prove resistant to therapy. For seborrheic keratoses, cure rates are high[2] and for thin seborrheic keratoses success is virtually guaranteed, but of course some will recur and new ones may appear nearby.

The other tumors and diseases listed in this chapter are suitable for treatment with cryosurgery only in some situations. It is important to realize that cure is not guaranteed and discretion is needed to avoid overzealous freezing of resistant lesions.

## PRINCIPLES OF TREATMENT
The majority of epidermal, warty lesions are easy to recognize and amenable to cryosurgery. Deep freezing is unnecessary and will produce unwanted side effects. It should be remembered that keratin is an excellent insulator so, when dealing with thicker lesions, it may be difficult to achieve subzero temperatures at the base unless the keratin is first debulked with a curette or scalpel before freezing. Seborrheic keratoses seem to "sit on the skin" surface and a good result is possible with little inflammation of surrounding or deeper tissues. Some viral warts, however, depending on the subtype of human papillomavirus (HPV) producing the lesion, have a deeper component, and considerable swelling and tissue destruction may accompany successful treatment. Some benign lesions with an increased melanin content, such as solar lentigines and labial melanotic macules, and vascular lesions often respond well, but those containing much connective tissue will be resistant.

There is great variation in susceptibility to the effects of cold and in some individuals blistering is seen after short, superficial freezes, whereas others may tolerate more prolonged or deeper freezes with only minimal edema. It is prudent to freeze cautiously at the first visit and to record accurately, in the patient's notes, the duration of freeze. This individual variation means that there are no hard-and-fast rules to determine the starting dose for a particular lesion. Table 8.1 gives average freeze times likely to be effective and the clinician must interpret these according to specific factors such as thickness of lesion, site and skin thickness.

On occasions there will be diagnostic uncertainty and it may be tempting to freeze a lesion on the assumption that its resolution would indicate a benign pathology. However, some early malignant lesions can almost clear with light freezes. When dealing with melanocytic nevi, there is some concern that cryosurgery might reduce the color so that any subsequent malignant change would not be recognized until a late stage. Any uncertainty should be resolved with a biopsy before cryosurgery. Also remember that verrucous thickening can be a feature of premalignant and malignant tumors.

## LESIONS TO AVOID
Although cryosurgery has been used to treat almost every conceivable skin lesion there are some situations in which it is generally best to avoid this approach. This is because either there are better alternatives or it could be detrimental. **Epidermal nevi** may initially respond to cryosurgery, but recurrence is the norm and these are better treated with full-thickness excision.[3] **Hypertrophic lichen planus** may become a little less itchy after long freezes and cryosurgery occasionally flattens lesions but the results are generally not better than high-potency topical steroids.

### Acne Cysts
In the past, gentle cryosurgery was used as a means to reduce early inflammatory and comedonal acne. Modern oral and topical antibiotic regimens and oral isotretinoin have reduced the need for cryosurgical treatments of acne. The advent of effective topical remedies has decreased the use of cryosurgery to treat inflammatory papules and comedones. Some deep nodules may respond to freeze–thaw cycles of 10–20 s.[4] Some superficial cysts appear rapidly and are disfiguring. Here a single freeze of 5–10 s may be sufficient and the results can be dramatic with complete flattening overnight (**Figure 8.1**). This outcome can also be accomplished with intralesional triamcinolone (2 mg/mL). There is a small risk of hypopigmentation with both treatments. Steroid injections may cause dermal atrophy if the concentration of the suspension is too high

*Table 8.1* Cryosurgery of Benign Lesions

| Name of skin lesion | Freeze time total (s) | Freeze–thaw cycles | Halo diameter (mm) | Method |
|---|---|---|---|---|
| Acne cysts | 5–10 | 1 | 0 | OS |
| Acrochordons – skin tags | 5–10 | 1-2 | 0 | OS or CT |
| Angiofibromas (adenoma sebaceum) | 10–15 | 1 | 0 | P or OS |
| Angiomas (cherry and spider angiomas) | 5–10 | 1 | 0 | P or OS |
| Benign lichenoid keratosis | 5–10 | 1 | 2 | OS |
| Chondrodermatitis nodularis | 10–20 | 1 | 1–2 | OS |
| Dermatofibromas | 30 | 1 | 2 | OS |
| Digital mucous cyst | 10–20 | 1 | 0 | OS or P after needling |
| Granulation tissue | 20–30 | 1 | 0 | OS |
| Granuloma annulare | 5–10 | 1 | 0 | OS |
| Granuloma faciale | 10 | 1 | 0 | OS (consider IS) |
| Hemangiomas (strawberry) | 10–20 | 1–2 | 2 | P |
| Keloids and hypertrophic scars | 20–30 | 1 | 1 | OS (with IS) |
| Lymphangioma | 15 | 1 | 1 | P |
| Molluscum | 5 | 1 | 0 | OS |
| Mucocele | 10–20 | 1 | 0 | P |
| Pearly penile papules | 10 | 2 | 0 | OS |
| Porokeratosis | 5–10 | 1 | 1 | OS |
| Prurigo nodularis | 10–30 | 1 | 1 | OS (consider IS) |
| Pyogenic granuloma | 20–30 | 1 | 1 | P or CT |
| Sebaceous hyperplasia | 5–10 | 1 | 0 | OS or P |
| Seborrheic keratoses: | 5–20 | 1 or 2 | 2 | OS |
| dermatosis papulosa nigra | 5–10 | 1 | 0–1 | OS |
| Solar lentigo | 3–5 | 1 | 0 | OS or CTA |
| Steatocystoma multiplex | 10 | 1 | 0 | OS |
| Syringoma | 5–10 | 1 | 0 | P or OS |
| Tattoos | 30 | 2 | 1 | OS |
| Venous lake | 5–15 | 1 | 1–1.5 | P |
| Viral warts: (common, flat, plantar) | 5–30 | 1–2 | 2 | OS |
| anogenital wart | 5 | 2 | 1 | OS |
| filiform wart | 5 | 1-2 | 1 | F or OS |
| Xanthelasma | 15 | 1 | 0 | P |

The times recommended either are from published literature or have been used successfully by one of the authors of this book. Freeze times are approximate and will vary based on the thickness, size, and location of the lesion.

CTA, cotton-tipped applicator; CT, Cryo Tweezer or forceps. IS, intralesional steroid; OS, open spray; P, probe.

(>3 mg/mL). Cryosurgery may cause temporary crusting of the treated cysts as an undesirable side effect. In our experience, patients tend to prefer the results of intralesional steroids over cryosurgery. Cryosurgery still has a role in the treatment of patients who are needle phobic. There may also be rare occasions when a pregnant woman, wishing to avoid any medication, will benefit from a 5-second freeze to a series of these lesions.

### Acrochordons – Skin Tags

Skin tags are common, benign, pedunculated tumors that occur predominantly in the flexural aspects of the body, and most often in overweight and older adults. Cryospray with a bent spray tip or small aperture tip is a fast and easy method to treat skin tags. One of the least painful and efficient techniques is to use Cryo Tweezers, which comprise a large Teflon-coated brass tweezer end that holds the cold temperature after being dipped into liquid nitrogen.

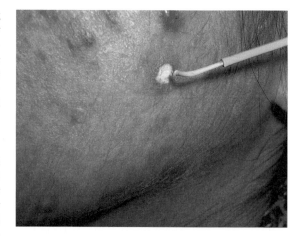

*Figure 8.1* **Acne cyst being treated with 5–10 seconds of cryosurgery. (Courtesy of Richard Usatine, MD.)**

The tags are grasped and held until the freeze margin reaches normal tissue at the skin surface (**Figure 8.2**). More details of this equipment appear in Chapter 3. Snipping or electrodesiccation can also be an effective method for treating skin tags, but cryosurgical methods do not require injections and cause no bleeding, and the discomfort is minimal. Cryo Tweezers are particularly useful on the eyelids where a spray can spatter nitrogen onto surrounding skin and risk entry into the eye. The best technique is to pull the tag and lid away from the eye to protect the globe from cryodamage (**Figure 8.3**), continuing the freeze until the whole tag is white to the base. Cryo Tweezers can be cleaned between patients using an alcohol wipe.

## Angiofibromas

Angiofibromas (adenoma sebaceum) are seen in the rare condition of tuberous sclerosis (**Figure 8.4**). The facial distribution makes them unsightly. Case reports describe good results with repeated cycles of cryosurgery[5] but long freezes are needed to remove the larger lesions and the risk of hypopigmentation is great. Laser therapy may therefore be a better choice. Angiofibromas may be seen in patients who do not have tuberous sclerosis and these smaller lesions (**Figure 8.5**) may respond well to a liquid nitrogen spray or contact probe.

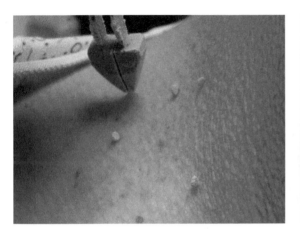

*Figure 8.2* Cryo Tweezers treating many skin tags on the neck. (Courtesy of Richard Usatine, MD.)

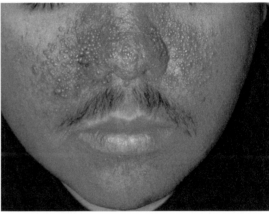

*Figure 8.4* Angiofibromas (adenoma sebaceum) on the face of a young man with tuberous sclerosis. Cryosurgery is one treatment option. (Courtesy of the University of Texas Health Science Center, San Antonio Division of Dermatology.)

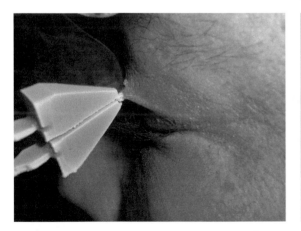

*Figure 8.3* Cryo Tweezers treating a skin tag on the upper eyelid. Note how the eyelid is elevated during treatment to avoid damage to the globe. (Courtesy of Richard Usatine, MD.)

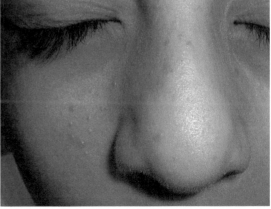

*Figure 8.5* Angiofibromas on the face of a young girl who does not have tuberous sclerosis. Cryosurgery is one treatment option. (Courtesy of Richard Usatine, MD.)

Patients with tuberous sclerosis also have periungual fibromas (Koenen's tumors) (**Figure 8.6**). Freezing the base of the lesion for 15 s is often enough to cause separation of the tumor from its relatively narrow base at the nailfold. Surgical excision is more likely to be successful in periungual fibromas that do not have a narrow base.

### Angiomas

Small vascular lesions such as cherry angiomas (senile angiomas, Campbell de Morgan's spots) and spider angiomas may respond to cryosurgery (**Figure 8.7**). All of these vascular lesions are best treated using a cryoprobe to compress the angioma during the freezing (**Figure 8.8**). No more than 10 s total freeze time should be needed, even for the larger lesions. Electrodesiccation and laser therapy are more effective methods of treatment and allow the clinician to see the final result at the time of treatment. Larger angiomas may be anesthetized and shaved off, and the base burned with electrosurgery.

### Benign Lichenoid Keratosis

A benign lichenoid keratosis may have similar features to cutaneous cancers so it is often diagnosed after a biopsy is performed (**Figure 8.9**). These lesions are also called lichen planus-like keratoses and show regression features on dermoscopy (pigmented granular pattern) (see Appendix C). They may represent an evolving or regressing seborrheic keratosis, and are easily diagnosed, histologically, with a shave biopsy. Once the diagnosis has been made, cryosurgery is an effective treatment option if there is any remaining lesion.

### Chondrodermatitis Nodularis Helicis

Chondrodermatitis nodularis helicis presents as a painful nodule on the pinna and is likely related to the pressure that develops on the ear while lying in bed (**Figure 8.10**). Initially people are advised to think of ways to reduce the pressure by using soft pillows, sleeping on the other side, fashioning a foam protective device, etc. In the event of failure, cryosurgery is one therapeutic option. It is crucial to make sure that the nodule on the ear is not a skin cancer before using any destructive method. If the ear nodule is clearly benign, there are many options for treatment. Freezing with a spray or probe for 10–20 s (consider offering anesthesia first) produces an inflammatory reaction that in some way leads to resolution of the condition in about 50% of sufferers. Additional treatment options include intralesional steroid injections and elliptic excision of the nodule, including removal of the inflamed cartilage.[6]

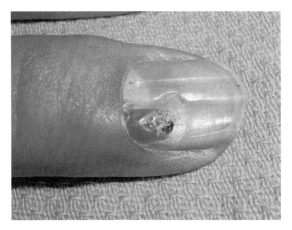

*Figure 8.6* Periungual fibroma (Koenen's tumor) on the finger of a man with tuberous sclerosis. Cryosurgery and excision are treatment options. (Courtesy of Richard Usatine, MD.)

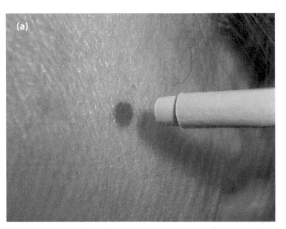
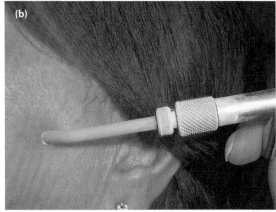

*Figure 8.7* Cherry angioma on the face of woman: (a) before cryosurgery; (b) treatment with a cryoprobe. (Courtesy of Richard Usatine, MD.)

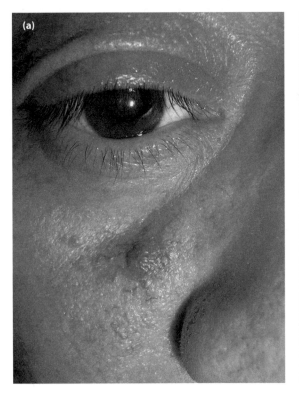
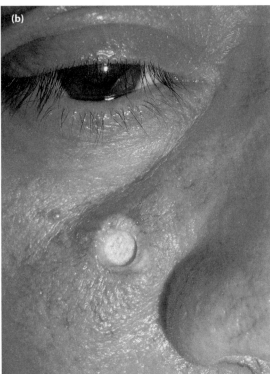

*Figure 8.8* (a) Spider angioma on the face; (b) spider angioma after treatment with a cryoprobe and liquid nitrogen. Note the indentation where the probe was used to compress the angioma. (Courtesy of Richard Usatine, MD.)

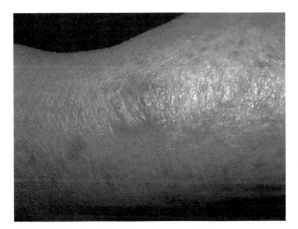

*Figure 8.9* Benign lichenoid keratosis (lichen planus-like keratosis) on the arm, proven by a shave biopsy. (Courtesy of Richard Usatine, MD.)

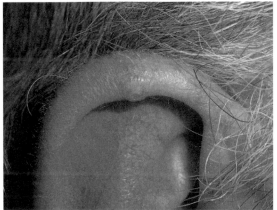

*Figure 8.10* Chondrodermatitis nodularis helicis: this is the most typical location for this inflammatory nodule. Treatment options include cryosurgery and excision. (Courtesy of Richard Usatine, MD.)

### Condyloma Acuminata (see Viral Warts)

*Dermatofibroma*

If the diagnosis of dermatofibroma is in doubt the nodule should be excised, but diagnosis is often possible by pinching the nodule and observing the positive dimple sign and noting the hyperpigmented halo and central scar-like structures (**Figure 8.11**). Dermoscopic findings are

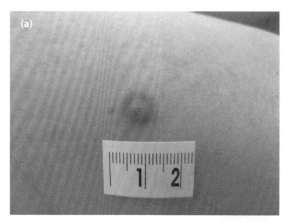

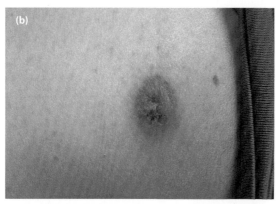

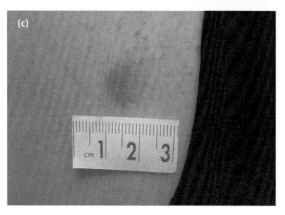

*Figure 8.11* (a) Dermatofibroma with hyperpigmented halo. (b) Blistering and erythema after treatment with cryosurgery. (c) Dermatofibroma that is flatter and partially depigmented after cryosurgery. (Courtesy of Daniel Stulberg, MD.)

also very helpful (see Appendix C). When the diagnosis is certain, it can be left untouched, excised, or frozen with liquid nitrogen. Certainly the nodular component can be flattened with cryosurgery but a pale area may be left behind (Figure 8.11). In one study each dermatofibroma was treated by liquid nitrogen cryospray for about 30 s to produce a visible freezing of the tumor and a 2-mm border of surrounding skin.[7] The overall response to therapy, as assessed by the patient, was excellent or good in 32 out of 35. The results assessed by an observer were excellent or good in 31 out of 35 lesions: 15 patients required 1 treatment, 16 patients 2 treatments and 4 patients 3 treatments.[7] A 30-s freeze time is the same aggressive freeze time used to treat basal cell carcinomas, and a local lidocaine injection should be offered for anesthesia before such treatment.

### Digital Myxoid Cyst (Digital Mucous Cyst)

Surgical excision, needle drainage, cryosurgery, and triamcinolone injection are all treatment options for a digital myxoid cyst (**Figure 8.12**). If cryosurgery is chosen it needs to be fairly aggressive in order to produce fibrosis in the walls of the cyst. In one study, 14 patients with myxoid cysts of the finger were treated with liquid nitrogen spray.[8] In order not to miss any tract to the joint, the field treated included the cyst and skin as far as the joint. Two freeze–thaw cycles of 30 s were carried out (note this is the same aggressive treatment used for a nodular basal cell carcinoma and should be performed with anesthesia). Twelve patients were cured without any permanent damage to the nail apparatus. No recurrences developed during follow-up for up to 3.4 years. There is considerable morbidity initially with significant pain and swelling.[8]

Another option is to numb the cyst or perform a digital block first, and then pierce the myxoid cyst multiple times with a needle. This will drain the viscous fluid and permit a less aggressive freeze of 10–20 s (**Figure 8.13**). Cryosurgery

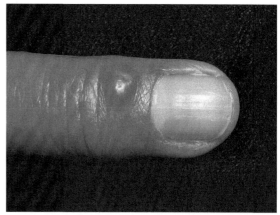

*Figure 8.12* Digital myxoid cyst (also known as a mucous cyst) in the typical location on the distal phalanx. (Courtesy of Richard Usatine, MD.)

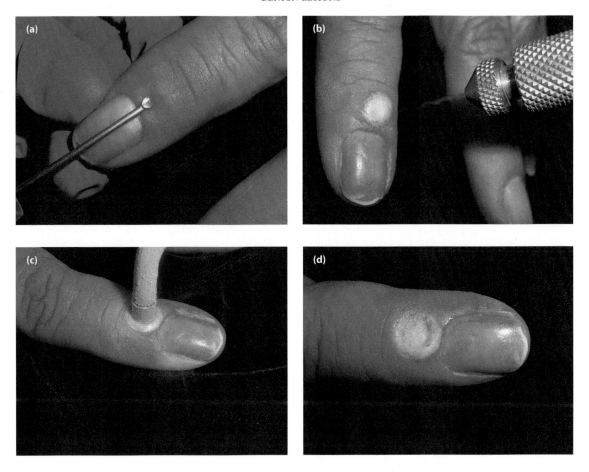

*Figure 8.13* (a) Drainage of gelatinous fluid from a digital mucous cyst using an 18-gauge needle after a digital block was performed. (b) Cryosurgery being performed with C-aperture tip. (c) Second freeze being performed with a cryoprobe. (d) Note the compression obtained with a cryoprobe for a deeper freeze. (Courtesy of Richard Usatine, MD.)

can be performed with a cryospray or cryoprobe technique. Surgical options include excision with an advancement flap[9] or a simple tissue-sparing approach described by Lawrence.[10] In this latter approach, a skin flap is raised around and under the cyst, and the base of the cyst is curetted and electrodesiccated. The same skin flap is sutured in place with excellent results.[10]

## Granulation Tissue

Cryosurgery as a treatment for granulation tissue can be highly efficacious and has been used in other specialties, eg after heart–lung transplantation granulation tissue at the airway anastomosis can become life threatening and is often treated by freezing.

Dermatologists encounter granulation tissue in several settings. Cryosurgery is effective in the management of hypergranulation in peristomal sites and in wounds healing by secondary intention (**Figure 8.14**). Although potent corticosteroid creams may be effective, the single application of liquid nitrogen is convenient (Figure 8.14).

When abundant granulation tissue forms around an ingrowing toenail with secondary infection or epithelialization, cryosurgery has been used by some clinicians. Using a spray, a single freeze of 20–30 s is carried out depending on the amount of granulation tissue present and the patient's pain tolerance. A second freeze may be needed at review 3–4 weeks later. This approach was repeated by another group and was thought too painful and ineffective to be recommended.[11] Ingrowing toenails are best treated with partial nail removal.

## Granuloma Annulare

Granuloma annulare is a benign granulomatous inflammatory dermatosis and can be resistant to treatment (**Figure 8.15**). At times it has been noticed that taking a diagnostic biopsy has led to resolution of a plaque. In the same way, the freezing injury induced by cryosurgery may bring about shrinkage or clearing of a plaque. In a study of 31 patients treated with a cryoprobe for 10–60 s all patients improved dramatically and in 80% this was after a single

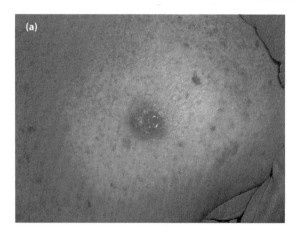

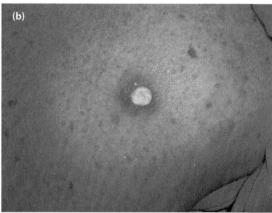

*Figure 8.14* (a) Granulation tissue remains after electrodesiccation and curettage of a basal cell carcinoma on the arm. (b) Cryosurgery with an open-spray technique was performed and the granulation tissue completely resolved. (Courtesy of Richard Usatine, MD.)

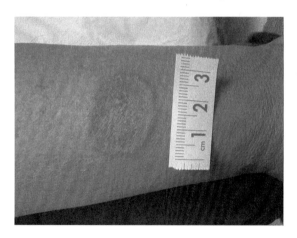

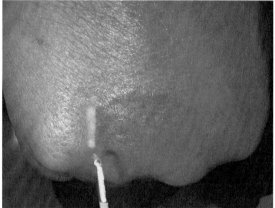

*Figure 8.15* Granuloma annulare with the typical ring of raised tissue. (Courtesy of Daniel Stulberg, MD.)

*Figure 8.16* Cryosurgery of granuloma annulare on the hand. The same patient had another lesion of granuloma annulare treated with intralesional triamcinolone. The patient and physician both judged the intralesional steroid as more effective 1 month later. (Courtesy of Richard Usatine, MD.)

freeze.[12] Although intralesional injections are our preferred therapy, if cryosurgery is to be used, we recommend shorter freeze times of 5–10 s to avoid significant pain, blistering, and post-inflammatory hyperpigmentation. In a single patient comparison study, intralesional injections with triamcinolone 5 mg/mL were more effective than cryosurgery (**Figure 8.16**).[13]

### Granuloma Faciale

Granuloma faciale is a rare disorder characterized by asymptomatic papules, nodules, and plaques on the face (**Figure 8.17**). Several medical and surgical methods have been used to treat it with variable results. Cryosurgery has been used as a sole therapy freezing the lesions for 10 seconds but also in one series of 9 cases the freezing was followed by corticosteroid injection. This was effective in all cases and apparently without recurrence.[14]

### Hemangiomas (Strawberry)

Strawberry hemangiomas in newborn babies can be treated with a cryoprobe applied firmly to the lesion with a contact gel interface for a period of 10–20 s. The aim is to allow the rim of ice to spread for up to 2 mm on to the normal surrounding skin.[15] Of course, cryosurgery is painful to the infant who does not understand the purpose of the treatment. It has the risks of hypopigmentation and scarring. Since the advent of oral and topical β-blocker treatment the use of cryosurgery for infantile hemangiomas has fallen out of favor. Oral propranolol has proven to be a very effective treatment. However, a small percentage of hemangiomas do not respond and cryosurgery remains

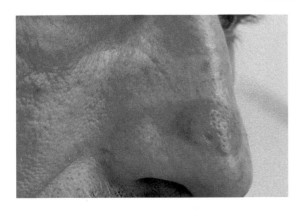

*Figure 8.17* Granuloma faciale on the nose. Treatment options include cryosurgery alone or combined with intralesional steroids. (Courtesy of Graham Colver, MD.)

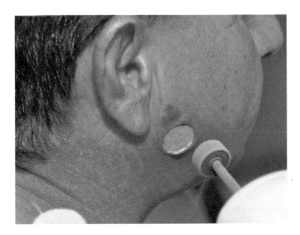

*Figure 8.18* Cryosurgery of a hemangioma using a cryo-probe with liquid nitrogen. Note the compression of the hemangioma after the probe was removed. (Courtesy of Richard Usatine, MD.)

an option for these lesions and others that have persisted into adulthood (**Figure 8.18**).

### Keloids and Hypertrophic Scars

Managing keloid scars is fraught with difficulties. There would be no need for the wide variety of approaches to treatment if any one of them was simple and effective. Cryosurgery is often a good approach but it may fail or need to be repeated on several occasions, and has significant side effects. Practitioners should be aware that once they have embarked on treating a keloid they become, in a sense, 'responsible' for it and the focus of the patient's frustration may now be directed at the clinician. This is important because the final outcome is often not ideal so realistic expectation must be part of the counseling. There are four approaches to the use of cryosurgery for hypertrophic scars

and keloids. In each of these, the cryogen may be used as either a spray or a probe except in the last case which utilizes a probe running through the scar.

1. Monotherapy with a success rate of 52%[16]
2. Cryosurgery + intralesional corticosteroids with a success rate of 75%[16]
3. Surgical debulking + cryosurgery
4. Intralesional cryosurgery.

*Monotherapy*

In 1982 the first report appeared on the relative resistance of collagen to freezing temperatures in the context of keloid scars.[17] Using two 30-second freeze–thaw cycles they found that, to achieve a useful result, over half the cases needed a second treatment. Even then the mean reduction in keloid volume was only 52%.[16]

More recently 30 patients were treated with two 15-second freeze cycles at 4-weekly intervals for 6 sessions.[18] The researchers found that there was significantly more flattening in younger lesions of less than 3 years' duration. Also younger lesions had an earlier response.[18]

Results from studies on earlobe keloids have been generally encouraging. Although the dosage schedules were not clearly defined, a group of seven young patients had one or more treatments resulting in complete resolution in five and a 25% reduction in volume in the other two.[19]

In summary, as a monotherapy it is wise to tackle small keloids only. The patient must be aware that multiple treatments may be needed. The method with a spray or probe is to freeze until a 1-mm halo appears on the surrounding skin. This may take as little as 15 s or considerably longer. It should be repeated every 4–6 weeks as necessary (**Figure 8.19**).

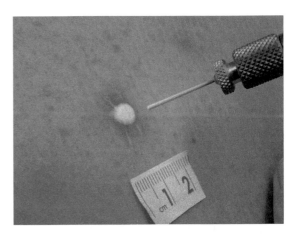

*Figure 8.19* Cryosurgery of a keloid using an open-spray technique. (Courtesy of Daniel Stulberg, MD.)

*Cryosurgery + intralesional corticosteroids*

Freezing the tissues to induce edema has been used as a method to facilitate the injection of steroid solutions (**Figure 8.20**). Many studies suggest that it is a better treatment than cryosurgery alone. Hirshowitz et al. reported complete regression (excellent response) in 41 of 58 patients subjected to combination therapy with a double freeze–thaw cycle using a cryoprobe followed by an intralesional steroid. They also found that keloid scars of the earlobes were the most responsive to treatment.[20]

A study to compare the efficacy of liquid nitrogen cryosurgery alone (double 30-second freeze–thaw cycle) with cryosurgery and intralesional triamcinolone (5 mg/mL) combination showed synergistic action of cryosurgery and intralesional corticosteroids.[21] Note that most lesions required 5- to 6-monthly interventions to produce excellent results. Combination therapy showed a significant objective response rate of 86.7% whereas the response rate was 70% with liquid nitrogen cryosurgery alone.[21]

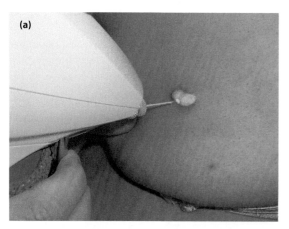

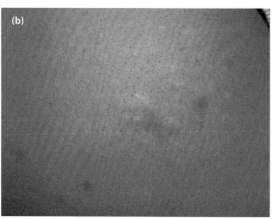

*Figure 8.20* (a) Cryosurgery of a keloid on the back before intralesional triamcinolone injection. (b) One year later the keloid was flat and no longer symptomatic from the single combined treatment. (Courtesy of Richard Usatine, MD.)

*Surgical debulking + cryosurgery*

Surgical excision with intralesional margins (ie not extending the excision lines on to normal skin) followed by cryosurgery to the base of the scar has been used by some authors.[22] It has also been suggested that the debulking should be performed after raising a thin "lid" from the top of the keloid, which is later sewn back in place.

*Intralesional cryosurgery*

This method involves the introduction of a hollow needle into one surface and its appearance at the other end. Liquid nitrogen passes through the needle, venting into the atmosphere while an ice cylinder or killing zone forms around the embedded part of the needle. Freezing can be assessed by the introduction of a thermocouple. Recent publications have suggested that the chief benefit of this technique may be shorter intervals between treatments as the exudates and swelling settle quickly.[23] Post-treatment healing times tend to be quick with less tenderness and less hypopigmentation.

In general, our preference for keloid therapy is to combine cryosurgery with intralesional steroids using triamcinolone acetonide 10–40 mg/mL after cryospray with liquid nitrogen. We do not use a double freeze–thaw cycle and freeze times are based on patient tolerance, not a set freeze time. Treatments are repeated monthly until the keloid is flattened.

Earlobe keloids respond well to surgical excision followed by intralesional triamcinolone so we rarely use cryosurgery for those keloids. Shave excisions with electrosurgery for hemostasis are rapid and the intralesional steroid is injected after excision while the anesthetic is still active. This rapid treatment produces immediate results and avoids the multiple visits that may be needed with cryosurgery.

## Lymphangiomas

Lymphangiomas are associated with underlying lymph dysfunction, but troublesome superficial areas can be improved with cryosurgery using a cryoprobe (**Figure 8.21**). Although lymphangioma circumscriptum may shrink somewhat with cryosurgery, the chance of complete resolution is small.

## Molluscum Contagiosum

This is a common viral infection that produces umbilicated papules which appear stuck on to the skin. Children are chiefly affected, particularly those with atopic dermatitis. The number of lesions present may vary from one or two to several hundred and they can persist for months or years. It is important to remember that the sudden development of large numbers of these lesions, in an adult, should raise the possibility of HIV or another cause for impaired immunity. Liquid nitrogen is applied until the surface of the lesion is white (**Figure 8.22**). This takes only 3–5 seconds. The central dimple, so characteristic

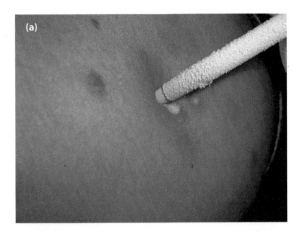

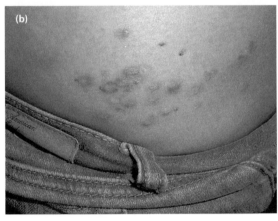

*Figure 8.21* (a) Cryosurgery of lymphangioma circumscriptum on the abdomen of a teenage girl using a cryoprobe with liquid nitrogen. (b) One month later the treated areas were flat and somewhat hypopigmented. (Courtesy of Richard Usatine, MD.)

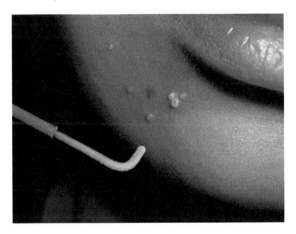

*Figure 8.22* Cryosurgery of molluscum contagiosum on the face of a girl. Note a bent spray extension was used for pinpoint accuracy and to minimize the pain of treatment. (Courtesy of Richard Usatine, MD.)

of molluscum, is highlighted. It is not necessary to freeze beyond the margin of the lesion. Over the next few days there may be temporary swelling then shrinkage and the papule falls off. Cryosurgery can rarely be used for children under the age of 6 years without the prior application of a topical anesthetic. After the first lesion is treated most children shrink away from any further attempts. EMLA may be applied at home or when the child first arrives at the office. For young children, less painful options include topical treatment with cantharidin, tretinoin, or imiquimod.

## Mucocele

These are alternately called a labial mucoid cyst or mucous retention cyst, usually presenting on the lower lip as a soft red or blue cyst up to 1 cm in diameter (**Figure 8.23**). They respond well to cryosurgery but larger lesions should be drained before application of the cryoprobe (Figure 8.23). Lubricant jelly may be applied first and the probe is pressed on to the lesion for about 10–20 s. If the cryoprobe is frozen first before contacting the lip, lubricant jelly is not needed. No lateral spread of ice is necessary. There may be considerable initial localized soft-tissue swelling, about which the patient must be warned, but the outcome is normally very good. Reports of 60% success after one treatment are usual but some studies have been even more optimistic.[24]

## Pearly Penile Papules

Pearly penile papules are symptomless, dome-shaped, flesh-colored papules occurring after puberty on the corona and sulcus of the glans penis (**Figure 8.24**). They are acral angiofibromas, which are often misdiagnosed as viral warts or sebaceous hyperplasia. They do not tend to disappear spontaneously. Various methods have been used and pulsed dye laser has its advocates but cryosurgery is quick and effective. Two cycles of 10 s with a fine liquid nitrogen spray is very effective and causes little morbidity.[25]

## Porokeratosis

Porokeratosis is a chronic disorder of keratinization producing papules and plaques with ridge-like borders known as cornoid lamellae. The most common variant is disseminated superficial actinic porokeratosis (**Figure 8.25**). New lesions may continue to appear for years and have a considerable cosmetic effect. No treatment is entirely satisfactory but cryosurgery is one approach that is often acceptable to patients despite the hypopigmentation that often follows. Short freezes of 5–10 s with a spray are best. The linear and Mibelli's variations of porokeratosis are no more amenable to resolution but a test area is always worthwhile. In one study, 18 of 20 porokeratosis Mibelli's lesions were successfully treated with a 30-second freeze.[26]

## Prurigo Nodularis

Prurigo nodularis is a chronic severely pruritic condition with "itchy bumps." It is seen along with lichen simplex chronicus in patients who find it hard to stop scratching their

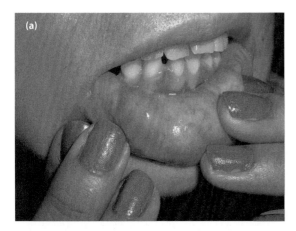

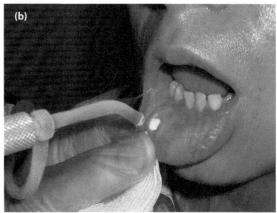

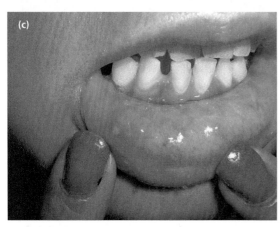

*Figure 8.23* (a) Mucocele on the lower lip. (b) After the mucocele was anesthetized and drained with a small snip excision, a cryoprobe was applied. (c) The mucocele is gone 1 month later.

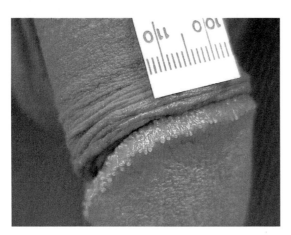

*Figure 8.24* Pearly penile papules around the corona of the glans. These can be treated with two 10-s freeze–thaw cycles. (Courtesy of Daniel Stulberg, MD.)

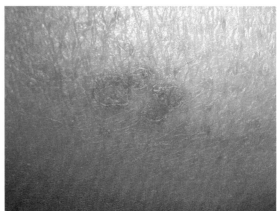

*Figure 8.25* Single lesion of actinic porokeratosis on the lower leg of a woman. Note the cornoid lamellae. (Courtesy of Richard Usatine, MD.)

skin (psychocutaneous conditions). Initial therapy often starts with high-potency topical steroids and oral antihistamines. The intensely itchy nodules of prurigo nodularis are well served by fine nerve endings so that the itching may resemble neuropathic pain. Medications to treat neuropathy such as gabapentin are often used for recalcitrant cases of prurigo nodularis.[27] Cryosurgery is known to create a degree of skin anesthesia and this property has been used to treat prurigo nodularis (**Figure 8.26**). In one case report, multiple freeze–thaw cycles with liquid nitrogen were used to create a blistering freeze for each nodule.[28] The freeze times varied from 10 s to 30 s. The lesions took weeks to heal and there was much initial hypopigmentation. The itching resolved, the nodules flattened, and repigmentation occurred over time.[28] Another treatment option involves using cryosurgery combined with intralesional injection of triamcinolone in a similar manner to keloids.

### Pyogenic Granulomas

Pyogenic granulomas respond to cryosurgery and can be treated with a probe or spray applied until the ice ball reaches the normal skin. Depending on the size this may range from 15 s to 45 s. It is wise to obtain tissue for histology if the clinical diagnosis is in any doubt. Prominent papular, nodular, or pedunculated lesions can be broken or curetted off while "iced" and sent for histology. Recurrent lesions may be particularly suitable for freezing, usually using no more than a single freeze–thaw cycle of 20–30s. Higher cure rates are likely to be obtained with a shave excision followed by curettage and electrodesiccation. However, this method always requires local anesthetic. Cryosurgery may be a good alternative in children who fear needles and may allow the use of a cryoprobe or Cryo Tweezers (**Figure 8.27**).

### Sebaceous Hyperplasia

Sebaceous hyperplasia is most often seen on the central face of older individuals and can be yellow and shiny, and resemble BCC (**Figure 8.28**). These benign lesions do not require any treatment, but several therapies are available including electrosurgery and trichloroacetic acid. If there is a suspicion of a BCC, then a shave biopsy sent for pathology is best. Cryosurgery can be used as a spray

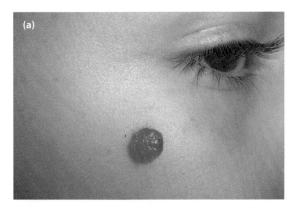

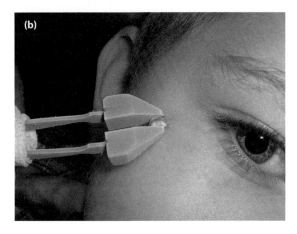

*Figure 8.27* (a) Pyogenic granuloma on the face of a young girl. (b) Cryo Tweezers are being used to treat the lesion. The young girl was afraid to be injected with local anesthesia in order to perform a surgical excision but tolerated the Cryo Tweezers treatment well. (Courtesy of Richard Usatine, MD.)

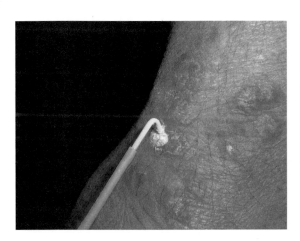

*Figure 8.26* Cryosurgery of prurigo nodularis refractory to medical treatment. (Courtesy of Richard Usatine, MD.)

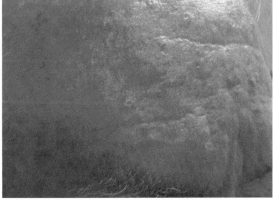

*Figure 8.28* Sebaceous hyperplasia on the forehead of a middle-aged man. Treatment options include cryosurgery and electrodesiccation. (Courtesy of Richard Usatine, MD.)

or tiny probe placed in the central depression for 5–10 s. Multiple lesions can be treated in quick succession.

### Seborrheic Keratosis

Seborrheic keratosis (SK) is a common benign tumor in adults and is seen with increasing frequency after the age of 50 years but may occur in the third decade. Single lesions may be seen but huge numbers may appear and this tendency is sometimes inherited. The clinical features are variable and skill is required to recognize all the variants. Dermoscopy is one of the best methods for the clinical diagnosis of the SK. Dermoscopic features include comedo-like openings, milia-like cysts, hairpin vessels, and a cerebriform pattern (see Appendix C).[29]

The most common appearance is a rough-surfaced plaque apparently "stuck on" the skin surface. Other features include a surface that may be "crumbly," dull, or resembling a "currant bun"; less often they are shiny. Reticular lesions begin life as a solar lentigo but slowly become palpable. Lesions on the face often start as solar lentigines. Pedunculated lesions have a narrow neck and are seen particularly in the axillae and inguinal region, and on the eyelids. Irritated or infected SKs may swell, redden, and develop deeper pigment, all of which can suggest malignant change. A shave biopsy may resolve the diagnostic dilemma.

Patients usually request the treatment of SKs for cosmetic reasons. Lesions may itch, be regarded as unsightly, or catch on clothing. Not uncommonly it is a grandchild tugging at or commenting on an SK that persuades a grandparent to visit the doctor. With increasing publicity about the early detection of skin cancer, more people now attend doctors with pigmented lesions, many of which will prove to be SKs.

Treatment by cryosurgery is effective and rewarding, although large and hyperkeratotic lesions are often best treated by curettage or shave excision alone. For standard keratoses up to a few millimeters thick, or for the pedunculated variety, liquid nitrogen can be used in much the same way as for viral warts. A spot freeze by cryospray is satisfactory and the usual method is to produce an ice halo of 2 mm (**Figure 8.29**).

If lesions with a large diameter (>1.5 cm) are treated by the spot-freeze method, the cryoinjury at the center may be unnecessarily deep. For this type the "spray-paint technique" can be used slowly moving the spray over the surface of the SK to effect an even distribution of freeze. Treatment times will vary widely according to size and thickness, but the usual range of freeze times may vary from 10 s to 20 s.

It is always best to err towards under-treatment, because SKs are not malignant lesions and hypopigmentation can be permanent if the freeze is overdone. With experience comes confidence in freeze times. Incomplete treatment often results in tissue remaining on the periphery (**Figure 8.30**). For this reason, the halo should be

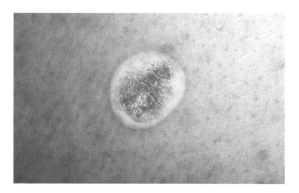

*Figure 8.29* Seborrheic keratosis after a spot freeze with liquid nitrogen as an open-spray technique. Note the 2-mm halo diameter. (Courtesy of Richard Usatine, MD.)

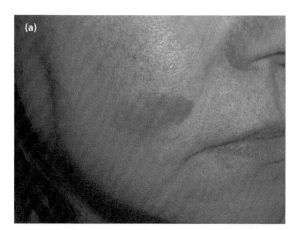

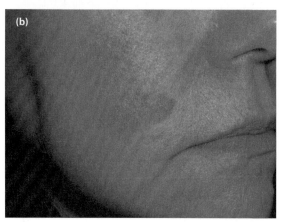

*Figure 8.30* (a) Large seborrheic keratosis on the face. (b) Some seborrheic keratosis remains on the edge after cryosurgery using a spray-paint technique. Note that there is no hypopigmentation or scarring, and a second treatment provided a full resolution with a great cosmetic result. It is better to under- than overtreat especially in cosmetically sensitive areas. (Courtesy of Richard Usatine, MD.)

symmetric around the whole lesion (**Figure 8.31**). If the thawing appears too rapid at one edge, just add a second freeze to that edge.

Some clinicians prefer to combine cryosurgery with curettage as a standard and feel that a light freeze renders the lesion easy to remove with a curette, producing an instant result and minimizing the risk of a persisting rim of keratosis.

One study compared cryosurgery with curettage for SKs in a group of 25 adults. They maintained the frozen area for 12 s after establishing an ice ball. The curettage was performed with a no. 15 scalpel. When assessed at 6 weeks and 12 months, approximately 60% of patients preferred cryosurgery and the difference was chiefly attributable to the need for dressings after curettage.[30]

*Dermatosis papulosa nigra*

This is a variant of SK, seen chiefly in people with dark skin, presenting as multiple small brown or black plaques around the cheekbones and eyes (**Figure 8.32**). The plaques may be flat or hang off the skin like a skin tag. Although light cryosurgery is effective for this condition the risk of pigmentary side effects is great. The most likely pigmentary change is hypopigmentation but hyperpigmentation can also occur.

Light electrodesiccation is a good alternative to dermatosis papulosa nigra (DPN) but, for patients who want cryosurgery, it is best to test the patient's response by treating a small number of lesions away from the central face (**Figure 8.33**). If the response is good and the patient is happy with the result, further cryosurgery may be performed. This is one instance when a written consent is important to document the informed consent process (see Box 6.1).

**Solar Lentigo**

Solar lentigines vary from light to dark brown and are seen on sun-exposed skin of the face and the dorsum of the hands (**Figure 8.34**). Patients may want these macules to be treated for cosmetic reasons, especially as they are perceived to be a sign of aging. Most importantly, before initiating any destructive treatment it is crucial to be sure that the brown macules and patches are not lentigo maligna or lentigo maligna melanoma. Dermoscopy can help differentiate the benign lesions from the malignant ones (See Appendix C). Both types of lentigines have moth-eaten borders on dermoscopy and should show no signs of malignancy such as rhomboidal patterns. If there is any clinical suspicion, a biopsy is warranted as the first step.

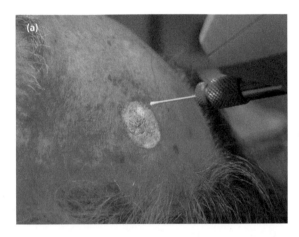

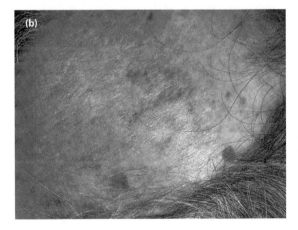

*Figure 8.31* (a) A large seborrheic keratosis on the forehead is being treated with cryospray using a spray paint approach and a 2-mm halo diameter. The green light indicates that the surface temperature is less than 0°C. (b) Large treated seborrheic keratosis resolved. (Courtesy of Richard Usatine, MD.)

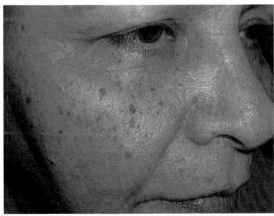

*Figure 8.32* Dermatosis papulosis nigra on the face of a 61-year-old Hispanic woman. Treatment options include careful cryosurgery or electrodesiccation. (Courtesy of Richard Usatine, MD.)

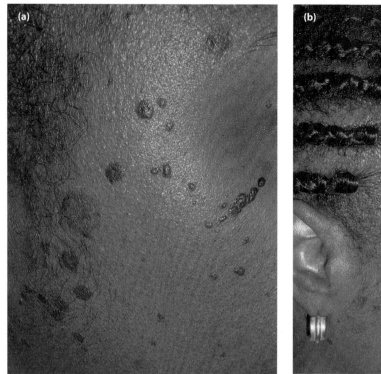
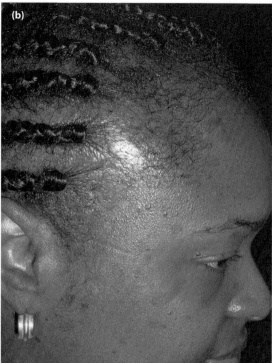

*Figure 8.33* (a) Dermatosis papulosis nigra on the face of a young African–American woman. Note that one large keratosis near the hairline was treated with non-aggressive cryosurgery to see how the patient's skin would respond. Although the lesion did not resolve, the patient decided to go ahead with further treatment, understanding the risks of hypopigmentation. She stated that she would prefer flat areas of hypopigmentation to elevated areas of hyperpigmentation. Patients' preferences and expectations are crucial to successful cosmetic treatments. (b) A happy patient after a number of cryosurgical sessions. Fortunately, any hypopigmentation was temporary. (Courtesy of Richard Usatine, MD.)

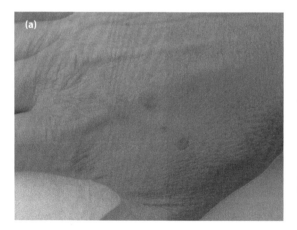
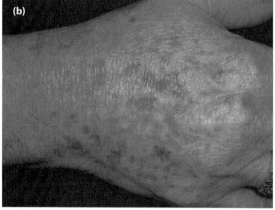

*Figure 8.34* (a) These hyperpigmented lesions on the dorsum of the hand could be solar lentigines, flat seborrheic keratoses, or flat warts. Regardless of the diagnosis, these lesions are amenable to treatment with cryosurgery with a single 5-s freeze. (Courtesy of Daniel Stulberg, MD.) (b) Many typical solar lentigines on the dorsum of the hand of a 52-year-old Hispanic woman. (Courtesy of Richard Usatine, MD.)

For benign lentigines, cryosurgery is one quick and effective treatment option (**Figure 8.35**). Other options include lasers, intense pulsed light, and topical trichloroacetic acid (TCA).

In one study, cryosurgery was compared with TCA for the treatment of solar lentigines on the dorsum of the hands. Liquid nitrogen was applied to the solar lentigines on one hand using cotton-tipped applicators for 3–5 s. For comparison, 33% TCA was applied to the solar lentigines of the other hand. Cryosurgery showed better results than TCA and this was especially true in lighter-skinned individuals. Cryotherapy produced more than 50% lightening in 10 patients (40%) compared with 3 patients (12%) in the TCA group. No patient experienced more than 75% lightening. Postinflammatory hyperpigmentation was the most common complication (40% and 44% of the patients with cryotherapy and TCA, respectively) and this was seen more often in darker skin types.[31]

In another study comparing TCA and cryosurgery using a "D" nozzle spray the freezing produced superior results. The device was held 3 cm from the lesion, and liquid nitrogen was applied for 1–5 s after initial freezing. Nine patients (47%) in the TCA group achieved more than 50% improvement compared with 15 patients (71%) in the cryosurgery group. Three patients in the cryosurgery group experienced more than 75% improvement. Lighter Fitzpatrick skin types also had better results, with 86% of the patients with skin type II achieving more than 50% improvement compared with 50% and 33% of the patients with skin types III and IV, respectively. Post-inflammatory hyperpigmentation, atrophy, or residual hypopigmentation was noted infrequently.[32]

Although the study using the cryospray technique produced better results than the cotton-tipped applicator, both methods of cryosurgery are acceptable.[31,32] Patients should be warned of the risk of post-inflammatory pigment changes. Meticulous use of sunscreen should be recommended after treatment of solar lentigines to avoid repigmentation and new lentigines.

The cryospray technique can be directed in a zigzag pattern to cover the lesions and 1 mm of normal skin at the periphery. If the edge is not treated sufficiently there will be a residual pigmented ring around what might be a relatively pale center and the contrast is cosmetically poor. If there are several lesions on the face it may be best to treat a test area in a less prominent site and assess the results after a month or two.

### Steatocystoma Multiplex

Steatocystoma multiplex can be a distressing condition characterized by multiple, asymptomatic, dermal cysts that usually occur on the trunk, face, and proximal extremities (**Figure 8.36**). The inner contents of these cysts appear like thick white toothpaste rather than the keratinaceous content of epidermal inclusion cysts (**Figure 8.37**). These

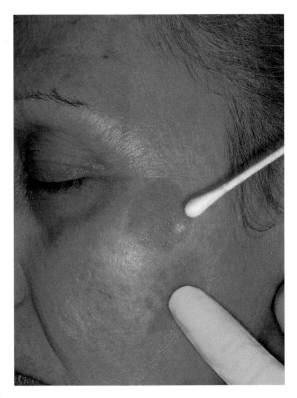

*Figure 8.35* Solar lentigo on the face being treated with a cotton-tip applicator dipped into liquid nitrogen. A gentle approach was used with an attempt to avoid hypopigmentation or increased hyperpigmentation. A gentle cryo-spray approach is also acceptable. (Courtesy of Richard Usatine, MD.)

dermal cysts may become infected and painful, and produce a visible exudate. Surgical drainage is often used but there has been some success with both oral retinoids and cryosurgery. In one case report a 10-second nitrogen spray was applied to non-inflamed lesions that were smaller than 2 cm. Six months after treatment, the cysts were flattened, leaving some hypopigmentation.[33] We recommend 10 s of cryosurgery with an open-spray technique as an acceptable alternative to surgery.

### Syringomas

These small benign eccrine-gland tumors are usually multiple and are found around the eyes (**Figure 8.38**). Many destructive treatments including electrodesiccation, laser, topical TCA, and cryosurgery have been tried with limited success. Syringomas are purely a cosmetic issue so the risks and benefits of any treatment plan must be clearly explained to patients seeking treatment. Cryosurgery may produce swelling in the soft tissues around the eyes and the usual risk of hypopigmentation should not be forgotten.

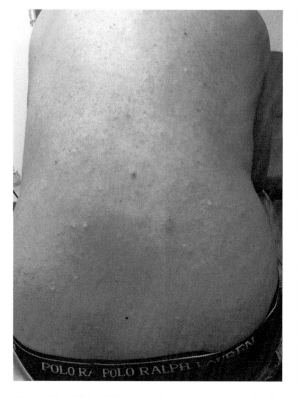

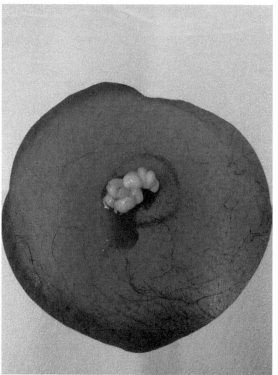

*Figure 8.36* Multiple lesions of steatocystoma multiplex in a patient with pachyonychia congenita. (Courtesy of Richard Usatine, MD.)

*Figure 8.37* Toothpaste appearance of the material drained from a lesion of steatocystoma multiplex on the chest. Alternately this lesion could have been treated with a 20-s freeze. (Courtesy of Richard Usatine, MD.)

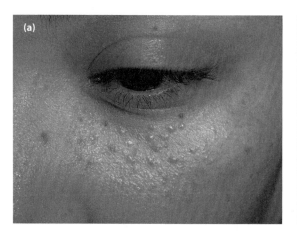

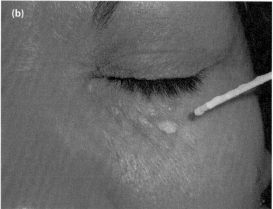

*Figure 8.38* (a) Syringomas under the eye of a woman. (b) Syringomas being treated with cryosurgery using a bent tip extension pointed away from the eye. (Courtesy of Richard Usatine, MD.)

However, treating a test area and waiting for a month to assess the benefit may be worthwhile. Freeze times of 5 s are suggested. Care must be taken to avoid getting liquid nitrogen in the eye by using a cryoprobe or an eye protector such as a tongue depressor.

### Tattoos

Although laser treatment is the most common treatment for tattoo removal, cryosurgery is one option (**Figure 8.39**). Two freeze cycles of 30 s with liquid nitrogen are needed. Local anesthesia before the cryosurgery

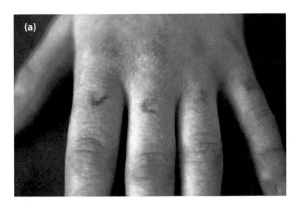
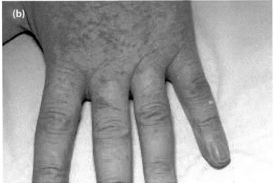

*Figure 8.39* (a) Tattoos can be treated by laser, surgery or cryosurgery. (b) One year after cryosurgery with two 30-s freeze cycles. The healing took 6 weeks after initial blistering in all lesions.

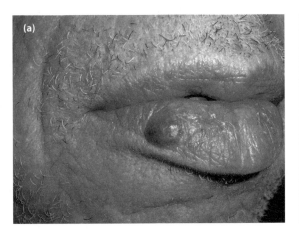
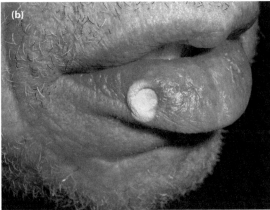

*Figure 8.40* (a) Venous lake on the lower lip. (b) Venous lake immediately after treatment with a cryoprobe and liquid nitrogen. (Courtesy of Richard Usatine, MD.)

is recommended. Patients need to be warned of the pain, swelling, and weeping of fluid that will occur in the first days after treatment. Healing times may be prolonged for weeks to months. However, some individuals are desperate to be rid of the tattoos and the stigma associated with them, and cannot afford laser treatment. For those individuals, cryosurgery may be a desirable option.

### Venous Lakes

The venous lake is a common variation of venous ectasia that occurs on the lip. It is not a hemangioma even though it may be called a "senile hemangioma of the lip." Venous lakes on the lip may be treated with liquid nitrogen using a cryoprobe or cryospray. The advantage of using a probe is that the lake can be compressed during cryosurgery in order to treat the deeper portion of the venous lake (**Figure 8.40**). In one published report of two cases, the venous lakes were treated with a cryoprobe that was precooled so that it did not adhere to the lip. A single freeze–thaw cycle was used

with excellent results visible in the published photographs. The authors recommended freeze times of 5–15 s depending upon the size of the venous lake. Halo diameters of 1–1.5 mm are suggested.[34] Alternate treatment options include surgery and laser therapy.

### Viral Warts

There are over 100 subtypes of HPV and many produce warts with different clinical features. As many warts occur in young children, the use of cryosurgery is limited by the inability of young children to endure the pain of treatment – indeed many young children fear cryosurgery even before the treatment starts. However, it remains a standard treatment option for older children, adults, and some very brave younger children.

A systematic review for the Cochrane Database analyzed 85 randomized controlled trials that have been published on treatments for viral warts.[1] A meta-analysis of cryosurgery versus placebo for warts at all sites favored neither intervention nor control. One trial showed cryosurgery to be better than both placebo and salicylic acid (SA) but only for hand warts. There was no significant difference in cure rates for cryosurgery at 2-, 3-, and 4-weekly intervals. Aggressive cryosurgery appeared more effective than gentle cryosurgery but with increased adverse effects. Two trials with 328 participants showed that SA and cryosurgery combined appeared more effective than SA alone (relative risk [RR] 1.24, 95% CI 1.07–1.43). None of the other reviewed treatments appeared safer or more effective than SA and cryosurgery. These findings demonstrate that cutaneous warts are difficult to cure regardless of the type of therapy used. Cryosurgery remains one option for treatment and these data do not dampen the enthusiasm of many patients who wish to be treated in this way. It is successful in some cases that have been resistant to topical solutions and it suits some people to have single treatments rather than protracted self-treatment. (See Chapter 7 for further discussion of the evidence on cryosurgery for warts.)

When cryosurgery and SA fail, intralesional candida antigen injections into all types of warts may stimulate the immune system to recognize the warts as foreign and eliminate the HPV infection.[35,36]

*Common warts*

These appear anywhere on the body but are most common on the face, hands, and knees. One option is a 12-week course of an SA-containing wart preparation. Cryosurgery is painful and may not be appropriate to inflict on a young child as first-line treatment. However, the application of local anesthetic cream (eg EMLA) 1–2 hours before therapy may be useful for some children. Markedly hyperkeratotic lesions can be pared down before freezing. When the redness and swelling settle, a few days after freezing, the patient may use an emery board each night before applying a wart solution.

In older children and adults it is often justifiable to freeze warts but it is wise to start conservatively and to document the time. If at the next visit there has been little reaction the freezing time can be increased accordingly. Cryospray with liquid nitrogen is very convenient. Initially a 1- to 2-mm halo of ice should be allowed to form on the normal skin surrounding the wart and this icefield maintained for 5 s. Some clinicians like to use a small ear speculum, a plastic shield with different apertures, or a neoprene cone placed over the wart (see Chapters 3 and 5). This technique ensures less damage to the surrounding skin for clinicians not comfortable with precise control of cryospray devices.

The bent spray tip on a Brymill cryogun is a great choice for cryosurgery of small warts and of any warts in children (**Figure 8.41**). The attenuation of the spray velocity and volume makes this technique less painful and less scary. This also allows the clinician to control the treated skin

more precisely and obviates the need for specula and plastic shields. If the cryospray is spreading out too quickly with a spot freeze, a pulse-spray technique is helpful to control the freeze-ball diameter.

Pedunculated and filiform warts can easily be treated with Cryo Tweezers (**Figure 8.42**). All of our patients prefer Cryo Tweezers treatment for pedunculated and filiform warts as it is less painful (probably because it affects less surrounding normal skin). For these reasons, this can be a great choice for treating warts in children as long as the wart is sufficiently raised to be able to apply the tweezers.

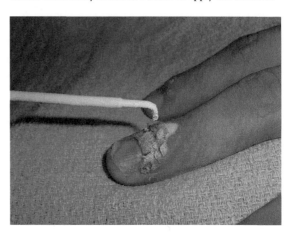

*Figure 8.41* Periungual warts in a young child being treated with liquid nitrogen. The bent tip extension is being used because the attenuated flow is less painful and scary for young children. (Courtesy of Richard Usatine, MD.)

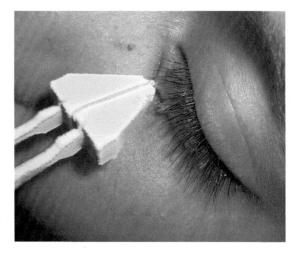

*Figure 8.42* Treatment of filiform warts on the lower eyelid of a young child using Cryo Tweezers. The child tolerated the procedure well. (Courtesy of Richard Usatine, MD.)

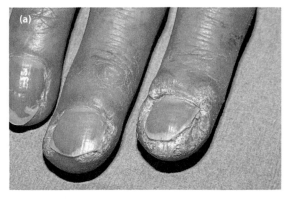

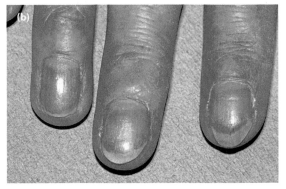

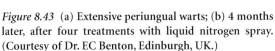

*Figure 8.43* (a) Extensive periungual warts; (b) 4 months later, after four treatments with liquid nitrogen spray. (Courtesy of Dr. EC Benton, Edinburgh, UK.)

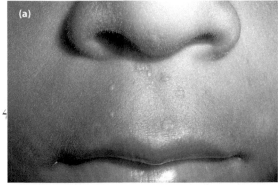

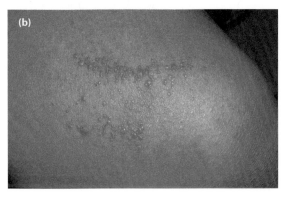

*Figure 8.44* (a) Flat warts on the face of a young child. (b) Flat warts on the leg of a 25-year-old woman that were spread by shaving.

Maximum success is achieved by treating warts at approximately 3-weekly intervals (**Figure 8.43**). Intervals longer than 6 weeks lower the cure rate and treating more frequently may not give time for the previous inflammation to settle down. If a wart is near a ring, it is essential to take the ring off before freezing because the post-cryosurgical swelling may make the ring too tight and act like a tourniquet.

### Flat warts

These are smooth, flat-topped, pink or brown papules often seen in large numbers on the face, legs, or back of the hands (**Figure 8.44**). Some are so small that they can be seen properly only with side lighting but they may persist for years and be cosmetically disturbing. Cryosurgery must be carefully considered because the large number of lesions and the risk of pigmentary change speak for a conservative approach by either avoiding treatment altogether or using the shortest of freezes (**Figure 8.45**). It is worth remembering that large numbers of flat warts developing suddenly (particularly on

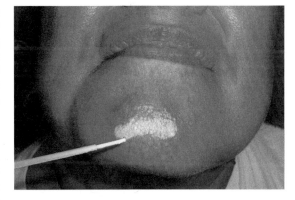

*Figure 8.45* Flat warts being treated with a superficial freeze using open spray with a spray-paint approach. (Courtesy of Richard Usatine, MD.)

the face) may be an early sign of HIV infection. Other treatment options include topical tretinoin, imiquimod, and 5-fluorouracil.

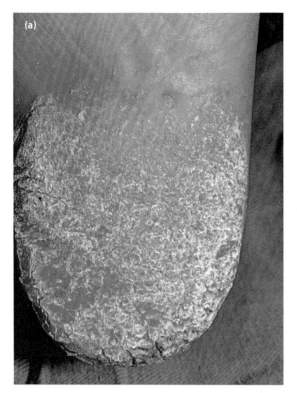
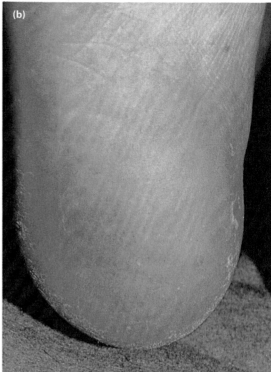

*Figure 8.46* (a) Large mosaic plantar wart; (b) 4 months later, after six applications of liquid nitrogen spray.

### Plantar warts

These warts on the soles or palms may be punctate, nodular, or mosaic (**Figure 8.46**). Pain is a problem particularly if the keratin builds up over weight-bearing areas. Epidermal ridges do not cross the verruca and this helps to distinguish them from corns. Also, the presence of black dots from capillary thrombosis helps to make this diagnosis. Cryosurgery is one option for treatment. Care should be taken so that the treatment is not so painful as to interfere with walking. Some clinicians prefer to pare down plantar warts before cryosurgery (**Figure 8.47**). In most studies a cryospray method was used.[37]

### Filiform or digitate warts

These are frond-like warts on the face, neck, and scalp of children and adults. They are particularly disturbing cosmetically when on the face. Fortunately this type of wart usually responds quickly to a short freeze to the base of the lesion. The Cryo Tweezers are perfect for treatment that is relatively painless (see Figure 8.42). A bent spray tip,

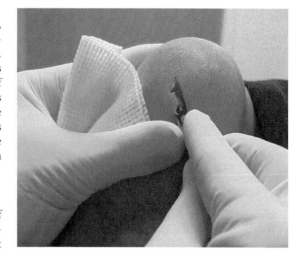

*Figure 8.47* Paring of a plantar wart using a no. 10 scalpel before cryosurgery. (Courtesy of Daniel Stulberg, MD.)

which can be rotated to any direction of spray, is ideal if a cryospray is being used for a lesion around the nasal vestibule or under the chin, because tipping the cryogen to an appropriate angle could lead to a rush of gas from the escape valve. A snip excision with or without local anesthesia is an alternate treatment option.

*Anogenital warts (condyloma acuminata)*

These may be associated with other sexually transmitted infections so it is crucial to test the patient for syphilis and HIV. These warts may respond well to cryosurgery. A long spray tip is helpful, including the bent spray tip or one of the long straight tips from Brymill (**Figures 8.48 and 8.49**). As for other warts, treatment should be repeated every 3 weeks until resolution. Topical imiquimod is one option to be used alone or together with cryosurgery. Massive anogenital warts may be best treated with surgery using a scalpel, razor blade, or electrosurgical loop.

## Xanthelasma

These fatty deposits around the eye may be cosmetically disturbing (**Figure 8.50**). They are often seen in patients with elevated lipids but can be seen in patients with normal lipid profiles. Treatment options for cosmetic purposes include: 50–70% trichloroacetic acid touched on to the surface, cryosurgery, and excision.

In one study of 100 patients with xanthelasma (237 lesions), closed-probe cryosurgery with nitrous oxide was used.[38] The investigators used 15-s freeze times and repeated the freeze–thaw cycles depending on the number and size of the lesions. Lid edema was observed immediately after the cryosurgery and remained up to 24–48 hours after the procedure, in all the cases. At the 6-month follow-up, 68% of the treated sites were clear. Another 6% of the cases looked clear except for pinhead-sized hypopigmentation in the center of the treated lesions. The remaining 26% of cases showed recurrence in the form of yellowish papules/plaques.[38]

In conclusion, cryosurgery can be effective but the lax nature of the skin at this site inevitably leads to marked edema for 1–2 days. Patients need to be warned of this side effect before proceeding with this treatment, regardless of whether liquid nitrogen or nitrous oxide is used as the cryogen. If liquid nitrogen is to be used, a cryoprobe technique is recommended.

## UNUSUAL INDICATIONS

Clinical practice is so varied that it is impossible, even in a specialist textbook, to cover the nuances of all the ideas, single case reports, and strategies that have been explored in cryosurgical practice. Experienced cryosurgeons will have had success treating unusual problems, in small numbers of patients, where other treatments have failed – but not necessarily report this in the literature. Some of these are now discussed briefly. Cryosurgery may cause significant damage to sensory nerves if used excessively but even after small doses there can be a minor sensory disturbance. This has been used to good effect in treating itchy conditions such as **lichen simplex** (10–20 s), **pruritus ani, pruritus vulvae**, and the itching associated with **lichen sclerosus** of the vulva. Freezes of about 10 s are suitable. In one small study of 12 patients with vulvar lichen sclerosus and severe intractable itch, 75% obtained symptom relief with cryosurgery, 50% for 3 years.[39]

Some rare vascular anomalies will respond to cryosurgery. **Angiolymphoid hyperplasia** is rare but unsightly and affects the head and neck but will shrink after cryosurgery.[40]

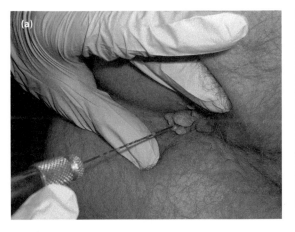 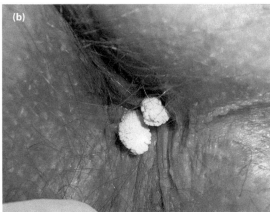

*Figure 8.48* (a) Perianal condyloma being treated with a long straight extension on a cryogun. This tip is perfect for work in the perianal area. (b) Condyloma acuminata that have turned white immediately after cryosurgery.

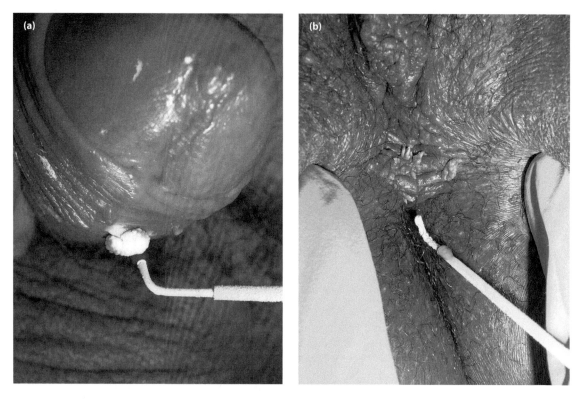

*Figure 8.49* Cryosurgery of condyloma (a) on the penis and (b) around the anus using a bent tip extension for accuracy of treatment and to minimize the pain. (Courtesy of Richard Usatine, MD.)

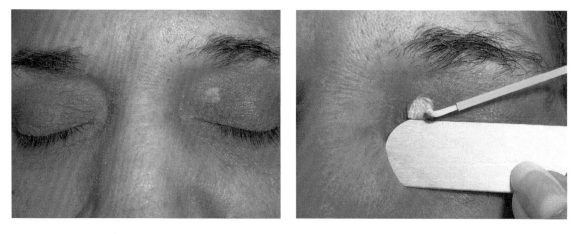

*Figure 8.50* (a) Unilateral xanthelasma on the left eyelid secondary to hyperlipidemia. (b) Cryosurgery with a bent tip extension while using a tongue depressor to protect the eye. (Courtesy of Richard Usatine MD.)

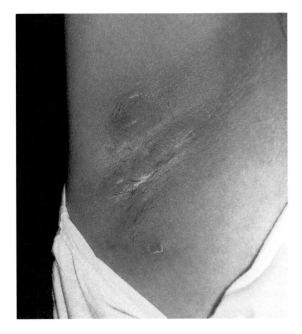

*Figure 8.51* Hidradenitis suppurativa: unfortunately most treatment options have limited effectiveness. Cryosurgery is one option for active cysts similar to intralesional steroids. (Courtesy of Richard Usatine MD.)

Inflammatory conditions such as **hidradenitis suppurativa** (**Figure 8.51**) may respond in certain circumstances. One small series reported the effects of a single spray cycle which achieved an intralesional temperature of −20°C. Eight of ten patients reported improvement without recurrence but it was painful and healing was slow.[41]

Infected conditions are not often treated but there have been reports of treating **orf**, especially at the early nodular stage.[42] **Cutaneous larva migrans** was, at one time, a target for cryosurgery but the side effects and very poor response rate have made this a less appealing option, especially now that we have good oral and topical anthelmintic medications. Cryosurgery for ***Leishmania donovani*** **cutaneous disease**, when the nodules are <1 cm, may be an alternative to sodium stibogluconate. It appeared to cure more than 75% of patients when applied for 2 × 20-s freezes at fortnightly intervals for one to four sessions.[43]

## CONCLUSION

Cryosurgery is extremely useful to treat many skin lesions with complete or partial resolution. It is relatively easy to apply in the office setting, usually with marked improvement in the cosmetic appearance of benign lesions. Liquid nitrogen spray is typically the fastest approach to treatment for most lesions, although other tools are available and effective as outlined in Chapter 4. For fluid-filled lesions, cryoprobes can compress the contents to facilitate freezing the deeper tissues to achieve the desired results.

## REFERENCES

1. Kwok CS, Gibbs S, Bennett C, Holland R, Abbott R. Topical treatments for cutaneous warts. Cochrane Database Syst Rev 2012;9:CD001781.
2. Herron MD, Bowen AR, Krueger GG. Seborrheic keratoses: a study comparing the standard cryosurgery with topical calcipotriene, topical tazarotene, and topical imiquimod. Int J Dermatol 2004;43:300–2.
3. Brandling-Bennett HA, Morel KD. Epidermal nevi. Pediatr Clin North Am 2010;57:1177–98.
4. Katsambas A, Lotti T. European Handbook of Dermatological Treatments, 2nd edn. Berlin: Springer Verlag, 2003.
5. Schepis C, Siragusa M. Cryosurgery: an easy and cheap therapy for facial angiofibromas in tuberous sclerosis. Eur J Dermatol 2010;20:506–7.
6. Devani A, Barankin B. Dermacase. Chondrodermatitis nodularis chronica helicis. Can Fam Physician 2007;53:821, 837.
7. Lanigan S, Robinson TWER. Cryosurgery for dermatofibromas. Clin Exp Dermatol 1987;12:121–3.
8. Dawber RPR. Myxoid cysts of the finger. Treatment by liquid nitrogen spray cryosurgery. Clin Exp Dermatol 1983;8:153–7.
9. Johnson SM, Treon K, Thomas S, Cox QG. A reliable surgical treatment for digital mucous cysts. J Hand Surg Eur Vol 2013 Oct 25. [Epub ahead of print.]
10. Lawrence C. Skin excision and osteophyte removal is not required in the surgical treatment of digital myxoid cysts. Arch Dermatol 2005;141:1560–4.
11. Masters N. Cryosurgery ineffective for ingrowing toenails. Br J Gen Pract 1991;41:433–4.
12. Blume-Peytavi U, Zouboulis CC, Jacobi H, et al. Successful outcome of cryosurgery in patients with granuloma annulare. Br J Dermatol 1994;130:494–7.
13. Usatine R, Smith M, Mayeaux EJ, Chumley H. The Color Atlas of Family Medicine, 2nd edn. New York: McGraw-Hill, 2013: 1026.
14. Dowlati B, Firooz A, Dowlati Y. Granuloma faciale: successful treatment of nine cases with a combination of cryosurgery and intralesional corticosteroid injection. Int J Dermatol 1997;36:548–51.
15. Bassukas ID, Abuzahra F, Hundeiker M. Regression phase as therapeutic goal of cryosurgical treatment of growing capillary infantile hemangiomas. Treatment decision, treatment strategy and results of an open clinical study. Hautarzt 2000;51:231–8.
16. Robinson JK, Hanke CW, Sengleman, RD, Siegel DM. Surgery of the Skin: Procedural dermatology. Philadelphia, PA: Elsevier Mosby, 2005.

17. Shepherd JP, Dawber RP. The response of keloid scars to cryosurgery. Plast Reconstr Surg 1982;70:677–82.

18. Barara M, Mendiratta V, Chander R. Cryosurgery in treatment of keloids: evaluation of factors affecting treatment outcome. Cutan Aesthet Surg 2012;5:185–9.

19. Fikrle T, Pizinger K. Cryosurgery in the treatment of earlobe keloids: report of 7 cases. Dermatol Surg 2005;31:1728–31.

20. Hirshowitz B, Lerner D, Moscona AR. Treatment of keloid scars by combined cryosurgery and intralesional corticosteroids. Aesth Plast Surg 1982;6:153–8.

21. Sharma S, Bhanot A, Kaur A, Dewan SP. Role of liquid nitrogen alone compared with combination of liquid nitrogen and intralesional triamcinolone acetonide in treatment of small keloids. J Cosmet Dermatol 2007;6:258–61.

22. Engrav LH, Gottlieb JR, Millard SP, Walkinshaw MD, Heimbach DM, Marvin JA. A comparison of intramarginal and extramarginal excision of hypertrophic burn scars. Plast Reconstr Surg 1988;81:40–5.

23. Har-Shai Y, Brown W, Pallua N, et al. Intralesional cryosurgery for the treatment of hypertrophic scars and keloids. Plast Reconstr Surg 2010;126:1798–800.

24. Ata-Ali J, Carrillo C, Bonet C, et al. Oral mucocele: review of the literature. J Clin Exp Dent 2010;2:18–21.

25. Porter WM, Bunker CB. Treatment of pearly penile papules with cryosurgery. Br J Dermatol 2000;142:847–8.

26. Dereli T, Ozyurt S, Ozturk G. Porokeratosis of Mibelli: successful treatment with cryosurgery. J Dermatol 2004;31:223–7.

27. Gencoglan G, Inanir I, Gunduz K. Therapeutic hotline: Treatment of prurigo nodularis and lichen simplex chronicus with gabapentin. Dermatol Ther 2010;23:194–8.

28. Waldinger TP, Wong RC, Taylor WB, Voorhees JJ. Cryosurgery improves prurigo nodularis. Arch Dermatol 1984;120:1598–600.

29. Marghoob AA, Usatine RP, Jaimes N. Dermoscopy for the family physician. Am Fam Physician 2013; 88:441–50.

30. Wood LD, Stucki JK, Hollenbeak CS, Miller JJ. Effectiveness of cryosurgery vs curettage in the treatment of seborrheic keratoses. JAMA Dermatol 2013;149:108–9.

31. Raziee M, Balighi K, Shabanzadeh-Dehkordi H, et al. Efficacy and safety of cryotherapy surgery vs. trichloroacetic acid in the treatment of solar lentigo. J Eur Acad Dermatol Venereol 2008;22:316–19.

32. Lugo-Janer A, Lugo-Somolinos A, Sanchez JL. Comparison of trichloroacetic acid solution and cryosurgery in the treatment of solar lentigines. Int J Dermatol 2003;42:829–31.

33. Apaydin R, Bilen N, Bayramgürler D, et al. Steatocystoma multiplex suppurativum: oral isotretinoin treatment combined with cryosurgery. Australas J Dermatol 2000;41:98.

34. Suhonen R, Kuflik EG. Venous lakes treated by liquid nitrogen cryosurgery. Br J Dermatol 1997; 137:1018–19.

35. Usatine RP, Pfenninger JL Stulberg, DL, Small R. Dermatologic and Cosmetic Procedures in Office Practice. Philadelphia, PA: Elsevier Saunders, 2012: 206–8.

36. Majid I, Imran S. Immunotherapy with intralesional *Candida albicans* antigen in resistant or recurrent warts: a study. Indian J Dermatol 2013;58:360–5.

37. Berth Jones J, Hutchinson PE. Modern treatment of warts: Cure rates at 3 and 6 months. Br J Dermatol 1992;127:262–5.

38. Dewan SP, Kaur A, Gupta RK. Effectiveness of cryosurgery in xanthelasma palpebrarum. Indian J Dermatol Venereol Leprol 1995;61:4–7.

39. August PJ, Milward TM. Cryosurgery in the treatment of lichen sclerosus et atrophicus of the vulva. Br J Dermatol 1980;103:667–70.

40. Wozniacka A, Omulecki A, Torzecka JD. Cryosurgery in the treatment of angiolymphoid hyperplasia with eosinophilia. Med Sci Monit 2003; 9:1–4.

41. Bong JL, Shalders K, Saihan E. Treatment of persistent painful nodules of hidradenitis suppurativa with cryosurgery. Clin Exp Dermatol 2003; 28:241–4.

42. Ocampo Candiani J, González Soto R, Welsh Lozano O. Orf nodule: treatment with cryosurgery. J Am Acad Dermatol 1993;29:256–7.

43. Ranawaka RR, Weerakoon HS, Opathella N. Liquid nitrogen cryosurgery on *Leishmania donovani* cutaneous leishmaniasis. J Dermatol Treat 2011; 22:241–5.

# 9 Premalignant lesions

This chapter deals with skin lesions that may progress to malignancy. They may be seen on mucous membranes, as well as on the skin, and as part of the nail apparatus. There is usually a protracted premalignant phase, but occasionally transformation is rapid. Actinic (solar) keratoses and Bowen's disease (squamous cell carcinoma *in situ*) are extremely common, have several clinical presentations, and are readily amenable to cryosurgery.

The important lesions for discussion are as follows:

- Actinic keratoses
- Actinic cheilitis
- Bowen's disease of the skin (squamous cell carcinoma *in situ*)
- Bowen's disease of the genitalia (including bowenoid papulosis).

## ACTINIC KERATOSES

These areas of adherent hyperkeratosis are the most common skin condition after acne and dermatitis. The lesions develop on sun-exposed skin, most typically at or after middle age. Fair-skinned people and those who live in areas of high sun exposure are more often affected, and for them their actinic keratoses (AKs) may appear at an earlier age.

### Epidemiology and Pathophysiology of AK

The prevalence of AK is estimated at 11–25% in adults aged more than 40 years in the northern hemisphere, and increases with age.[1] AKs have the potential to become squamous cell carcinoma (SCC). The rate of malignant transformation has been variably estimated, but is probably no greater than 6% per AK over a 10-year period.[2] In a large prospective cohort study, the risk of progression of AK to primary SCC (invasive or *in situ*) was 0.60% at 1 year and 2.57% at 4 years. Approximately 65% of all primary SCCs and 36% of all primary basal cell carcinomas (BCCs) diagnosed in the study arose in lesions that previously were diagnosed clinically as AKs. Many AKs did resolve spontaneously: 55% of AKs that were followed clinically were not present at 1 year and 70% were not present at the 5-year follow-up.[3]

### Morphology of AK

Actinic keratoses often begin as almost indiscernible telangiectatic areas with scaling. They may have this appearance for many months with little or no scale (**Figure 9.1**).

However, adherent keratotic scale almost always develops. The sites more often affected are the backs of the hands, forearms, and upper face. Several morphological varieties may develop, the main ones being:

- Common (**Figure 9.2**)
- Pigmented (**Figure 9.3**)
- Cutaneous horn (**Figure 9.4**).

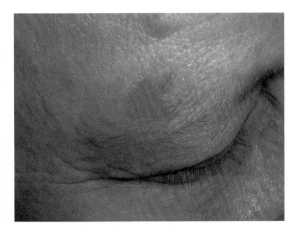

*Figure 9.1* Actinic keratosis over the eyebrow with prominent vascular pattern and little visible scale. (Courtesy of Richard Usatine, MD.)

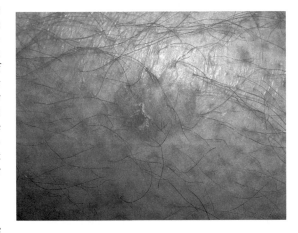

*Figure 9.2* Common actinic keratosis on the arm with white rough scale. (Courtesy of Richard Usatine, MD.)

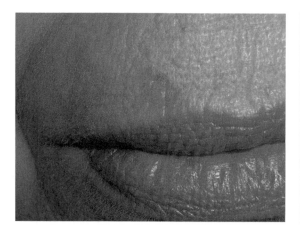

*Figure 9.3* Pigmented actinic keratosis over the lip that was biopsy proven to rule out malignancy. (Courtesy of Richard Usatine, MD.)

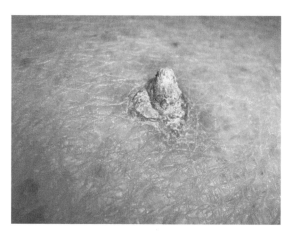

*Figure 9.4* Cutaneous horn resulting from an actinic keratosis on the leg of an older white woman. (Courtesy of Richard Usatine, MD.)

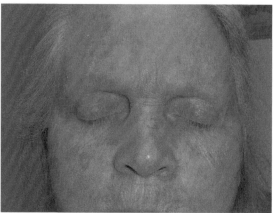

*Figure 9.5* Many actinic keratoses on the face that feel similar to sandpaper. The most advanced actinic keratoses were treated with cryosurgery and the remainder of the face was treated with 5-fluorouracil. This field treatment was successful. The patient has not had a single cutaneous malignancy to date with years of follow-up. (Courtesy of Richard Usatine, MD.)

### Common

Yellow or white rough scale is the main feature of this variety (Figure 9.2). The AKs are frequently multiple, with the overall effect being described as similar to touching sandpaper (**Figure 9.5**). In fact, touching the skin for areas of rough spots is an important aspect of a good exam to detect AKs.

### Pigmented

This type may be almost flat, and the pigmentation raises doubts, because it could be a melanocytic lesion. However, the typical scaly roughness is almost always present on pigmented AKs. If doubt exists then biopsy or excision is required rather than cryosurgery (**Figure 9.6**).

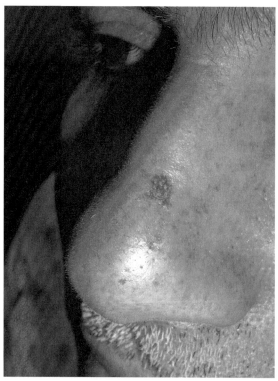

*Figure 9.6* Pigmented actinic keratosis on the nose that should be biopsied rather than treated blindly with cryosurgery. The risk of an undiagnosed skin cancer is too high for this lesion. (Courtesy of Richard Usatine, MD.)

*Cutaneous horn*

The primary pathology at the base of a cutaneous horn may be an AK, a viral wart, a seborrheic keratosis, a keratoacanthoma, or a squamous cell carcinoma (**Figure 9.7**). Features that may indicate malignant change are an indurated base and rapid growth (**Figure 9.8**). A deep shave biopsy, including the base of the cutaneous horn, is recommended before or instead of cryosurgery (**Figure 9.9**).

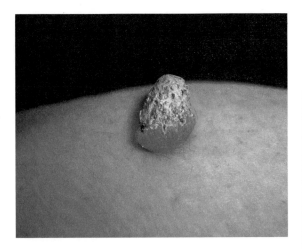

*Figure 9.7* Cutaneous horn arising in a wart. This lesion could also have been a keratoacanthoma but a shave biopsy provided evidence that this lesion arose in a common wart. (Courtesy of Richard Usatine, MD.)

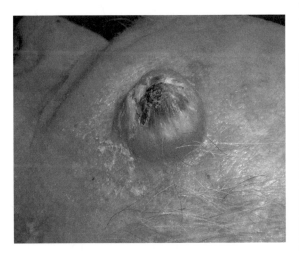

*Figure 9.8* Large keratoacanthoma on the forehead with central cutaneous horn. This is not an appropriate lesion for cryosurgery and treatment must start with a biopsy for histopathology. (Courtesy of Richard Usatine, MD.)

**Biopsy**

AKs are diagnosed clinically without a biopsy in most cases. A biopsy should be undertaken in the following situations:

- Thick lesions, particularly if there has been rapid growth (**Figure 9.10**)
- Lesions that show any other features suggestive of an SCC (cutaneous horn, bleeding, significant pain, larger size) (**Figure 9.11**)
- Pigmented AKs if there is any suspicion for melanoma (see Figure 9.6)
- Lesions that were diagnosed as AKs clinically but have failed to respond to cryotherapy of other local treatment.

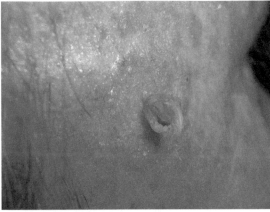

*Figure 9.9* Cutaneous horn arising in a squamous cell carcinoma in situ found in the area of the temple. (Courtesy of Richard Usatine, MD.)

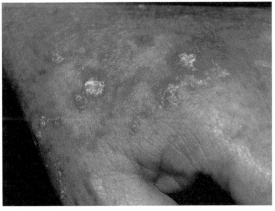

*Figure 9.10* Actinic keratoses on the back of the hand with some thicker lesions concerning for Bowen's disease. (Courtesy of Richard Usatine, MD.)

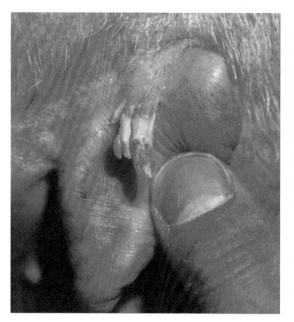

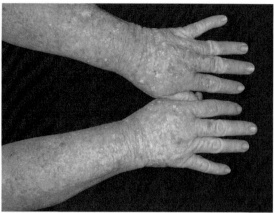

*Figure 9.12* Many actinic keratoses covering both fore-arms. The driver's side arm on the left had more actinic keratoses. This patient was treated with 5-fluorouracil after selective cryosurgery of the most advanced actinic keratoses. (Courtesy of Richard Usatine, MD.)

*Figure 9.11* Cutaneous horn arising in a squamous cell carcinoma on the ear.

A shave biopsy is fast and adequate for most lesions. If a deeper biopsy is needed of a thicker lesion, a deep shave or punch biopsy may be obtained.

## Management of AKs

Although cryosurgery is the quickest and most conveni-ent treatment of AKs in the office, there are many other adjunctive and alternate treatments (including those applied by the patient at home):

- Moisturizers should be used and sun exposure avoided in patients with dry, sun-exposed skin. No therapy or the application of an emollient is a reasonable option for mild AKs[4] – strength of recommendation (SOR) A.
- Sunscreen applied twice daily for 7 months may pro-tect against development of AKs[4] – SOR A
- Treat multiple AKs of the face, scalp, forearms, and hands topically with 5-fluorouracil (5-FU), imiqui-mod, or diclofenac[1,4] – SOR A (**Figure 9.12**).
- Topical 5-FU is an efficient therapeutic method and may be used for treatment of isolated, as well as large, areas of AK. It may be applied by the patient, and is inexpensive compared with other topical modalities[1] – SOR A (**Figure 9.13**).
- 5-FU cream used twice daily for 3–6 weeks is effec-tive for up to 12 months in the clearance of most AKs[4] – SOR A.
- Diclofenac gel applied twice daily for 10–12 weeks has moderate efficacy with low morbidity in mild

AKs[4] – SOR B. There are few follow-up data to indi-cate the duration of benefit.[4] In one study, diclofenac 3% gel was as effective as 5-FU cream for AK of the face and scalp, and diclofenac produced fewer signs of inflammation.[5]

- Imiquimod 5% cream has been demonstrated to be effective over a 16-week course of treatment, but studies have only measured 8 weeks of follow-up[4] – SOR B. By weight, it is 19 times the cost of 5-FU. They have similar side effects.[4] Imiquimod applied topically for 12–16 weeks produced complete clear-ance of AKs in 50% of patients compared with 5% with vehicle (number needed to treat [NNT] = 2.2). Adverse events included erythema (27%), scab-bing or crusting (21%), flaking (9%), and erosions (6%) (number needed to harm [NNH] = 3.2–5.9).[6] A major limiting factor is that it is approved for only 25 cm$^2$ of the face or scalp.
- Topical tretinoin has some efficacy on the face, with partial clearance of AKs, but may need to be used for up to a year at a time to optimize benefit[4] – SOR B.
- Photodynamic therapy (PDT) was effective in up to 91% of AKs in trials comparing it with cryotherapy, with consistently good cosmetic results. It may be particularly good for superficial and confluent AKs, but is likely to be more expensive than most other therapies. It is of particular value where AKs are numerous or when located at sites of poor healing, such as the lower leg[4] – SOR B.
- Ingenol mebutate (Picato): a short 2–3 days of treat-ment with daily topical ingenol mebutate from the sap of the *Euphorbia peplus* plant showed promis-ing efficacy, with a favorable safety profile in several

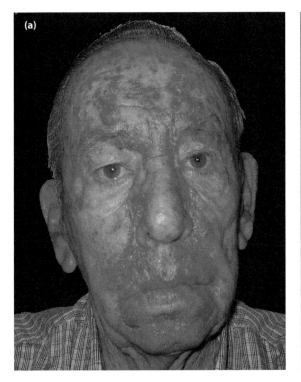
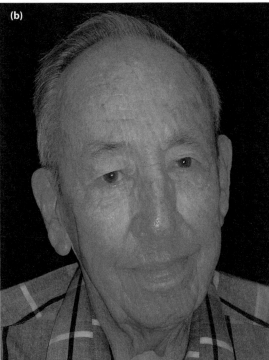

*Figure 9.13* (a) Actinic keratoses lighting up with erythema during the course of treatment with 5-fluorouracil. (b) Clear skin on the face 1 month later. (Courtesy of Richard Usatine, MD.)

randomized controlled trials (RCTs). One multicenter RCT showed 34.1–42.2% complete clearance of AKs with ingenol mebutate gel 0.05% for trunk and extremities, and 0.015% for face.[7] Another RCT with 0.05% gel showed a complete clearance of 71% of treated lesions.[8] A major limiting factor is that it is approved for only up to 25 cm² (this does not even cover one forearm).

## Cryosurgery

AKs are most often treated by cryosurgery using liquid nitrogen (**Figure 9.14**). It is simple, rapid, and inexpensive, and may be used as first-line treatment[1] (SOR C). One meta-analysis showed a 2-month cure rate of 97.0% with 2.1% recurrences in 1 year.[9]

Treating AKs with liquid nitrogen using a 1-mm halo freeze with a cryospray demonstrated a complete response of 39% for freeze times of less than 5 s, 69% for freeze times greater than 5 s, and 83% for freeze times greater than 20 s.[10] There is considerably more hypopigmentation caused by 20 s of freeze time.

The length of the freeze time should be based on the size and thickness of the lesion, using sufficient time for clearance while attempting to avoid hypopigmentation and scarring (SOR B). A cryospray method with liquid nitrogen is preferred over a probe method which could leave an imprint of the probe on the treated skin. The cryospray is easier to configure to the size and shape of the AKs which do not often come as conveniently round (**Figures 9.14 and 9.15**).

Fortunately, with good lighting and close inspection, the edge of each AK becomes more visible as the lesion begins to turn white with freezing (**Figure 9.16**). When freezing is started, and as the ice becomes established and the edge of the lesion clearer, the size of the lesion may turn out initially to be larger than considered clinically. It is important to freeze the total lesion with about a 1- to 2-mm "clear" edge. The total freeze time depends on thickness and size, and should be about 5–10 s based on existing data.[10] In my experience, some very thin early AKs may be treated with 3–5 s only.

Lesions up to 1 cm diameter can be treated by the spot-freeze method (see Chapter 5), using a freeze time sufficient to ensure adequate ice formation in the total lesion. However, larger circular or irregularly shaped lesions may be treated with a circular or paint-spray technique to 1–2 mm beyond the edge of the lesion.

### Spray tips

The bent tip spray devices are a particularly gentle method for cryosurgery of AKs around sensitive areas of the face

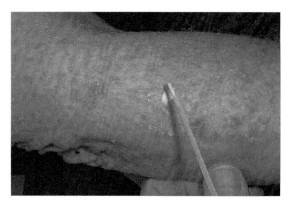

*Figure 9.14* **Cryosurgery of actinic keratoses on the arm using a bent spray tip. (Courtesy of Richard Usatine, MD.)**

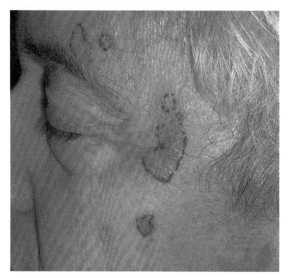

*Figure 9.15* **Multiple actinic keratoses on the left face in a man who drove for a living (in the USA). (Courtesy of Richard Usatine, MD.)**

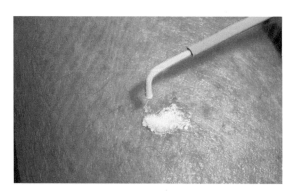

*Figure 9.16* **Cryosurgery of an actinic keratosis showing how the border becomes more visible during ice-ball formation. (Courtesy of Richard Usatine, MD.)**

(**Figure 9.17**). The 90° angle and the small aperture allow for a less shocking and less rapid flow of liquid nitrogen to the skin. However, the slower less exuberant flow of liquid nitrogen to the skin may require slightly longer freeze times than with a straight tip device. The bent tip can also be angled away from the eye when working on eyelids. The C-tip aperture is also a good choice for cryospray of AKs. A tongue depressor held over the closed eye is one way of protecting the eye when working near the eyelids.

*Patient selection*

Initially, it is important to choose the correct lesions for cryosurgery. The site and other factors will also determine whether this is the most appropriate modality. There are several points in favor of freezing:

- All ages can be treated, even patients in poor health.
- White people (Fitzpatrick skin types I–III) respond particularly well as a group because hypopigmentation and hypertrophic scar formation are less of a problem.
- It is safe to use even in high-risk sites for keloids.
- It is safe in those taking anticoagulants or allergic to local anesthetic.
- Lesions on sites with poor skin mobility (over the tibia) may be difficult to excise, but can be frozen safely.
- It can be used on skin that has previously undergone irradiation.

## ACTINIC CHEILITIS

Intense and prolonged exposure to ultraviolet light may lead to changes on the lower lip (**Figure 9.18**). This begins with dryness and then thickened white plaques start to develop. Variable inflammation and crusting follow.

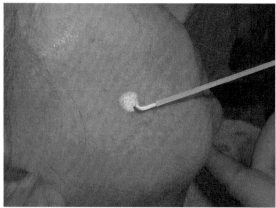

*Figure 9.17* **Cryosurgery on the face using a bent tip probe to minimize the pain during freezing.**

Actinic cheilitis should be differentiated from SCC, lichen planus, contact dermatitis, and lupus erythematosus. If the clinical picture is not clearly actinic cheilitis, then a shave biopsy should be performed.

Actinic cheilitis may be treated by cryosurgery using a single 5- to 10-second freeze–thaw cycle. No margin is needed. The time is based on how advanced the actinic cheilitis is and how much the patient can tolerate in a single freeze. In my experience, most patients cannot tolerate more than 10 s of freeze on the lip without anesthesia. If the patient pulls away early, a second freeze may be applied to reach the total time intended for the full freeze. Liquid nitrogen applied to the lip is usually painful and unpleasant for most patients. This is where the bent tip sprays and smaller aperture spray tips can be particularly helpful (**Figure 9.19**).

It is best to set up a follow-up appointment in 3–4 weeks to see if the treatment cleared the disease. A second cryosurgical procedure is reasonable if the first one was not sufficiently aggressive because the patient did not tolerate the freezing well. Another follow-up visit should be scheduled. At this time, if presumed actinic cheilitis did not respond to cryosurgery a biopsy is needed to avoid missing SCC, which needs more aggressive treatment including surgical excision.

## BOWEN'S DISEASE

Bowen's disease is also known as SCC *in situ*. The lesions begin as areas of pink, scaly, or crusted skin that have a slow radial growth pattern (**Figures 9.20 and 9.21**). The cellular

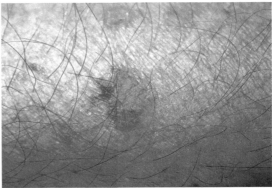

*Figure 9.20* The middle lesion is Bowen's disease (squamous cell carcinoma in situ) and the upper lesion was an actinic keratosis. Both biopsy proven on this man's arm. (Courtesy of Richard Usatine, MD.)

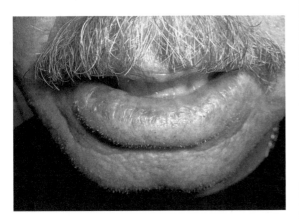

*Figure 9.18* Actinic cheilitis on the lower lip with erythema and scale.

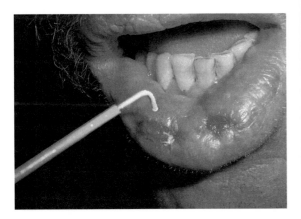

*Figure 9.19* Actinic cheilitis being treated after selected shave biopsies demonstrated that this was not invasive squamous cell carcinoma. (Courtesy of Richard Usatine, MD.)

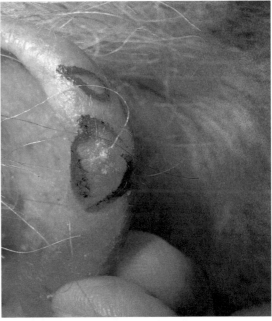

*Figure 9.21* Biopsy-proven Bowen's disease on the ear. (Courtesy of Richard Usatine, MD.)

changes are neoplastic, but localized entirely within the epidermis. When the changes breach the basement membrane, the lesion has undergone malignant transformation into an SCC. Bowen's disease is often seen on the leg below the knee in women with fair skin (**Figures 9.22 and 9.23**).

Table 9.1 compares and summarizes the main treatment options for Bowen's disease.

The risk of progression to invasive cancer is approximately 3%. This risk is greater in genital Bowen's disease,

and particularly in perianal Bowen's disease. A high risk of recurrence, including late recurrence, is a particular feature of perianal Bowen's disease and prolonged follow-up is recommended for this variant[11] – SOR A.

There is reasonable evidence to support the use of 5-FU[11] – SOR B. It is more practical than surgery for large lesions, especially at potentially poor healing sites, and has been used for "control" rather than cure in some patients with multiple lesions.[11]

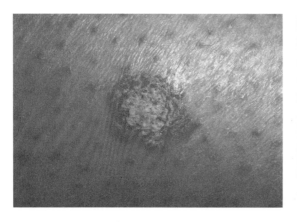

*Figure 9.22* Bowen's disease on the lower leg of a woman with erythema and scale. (Courtesy of Richard Usatine, MD.)

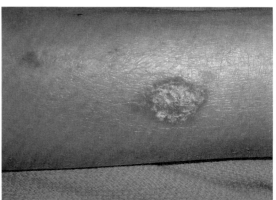

*Figure 9.23* Bowen's disease on the lower leg of a woman showing significant scale and a well-demarcated border. (Courtesy of Richard Usatine, MD.)

*Table 9.1* Summary of the Main Treatment Options for Bowen's Disease[11]

| Lesion characteristics | Topical 5-FU | Topical imiquimod[a] | Cryotherapy | Curettage | Excision | PDT | Radiotherapy | Laser[b] |
|---|---|---|---|---|---|---|---|---|
| Small, single/few, good healing site[c] | 4 | 3 | 2 | 1 | 3 | 3 | 5 | 4 |
| Large, single, good healing site[c] | 3 | 3 | 3 | 5 | 5 | 2 | 4 | 7 |
| Multiple, good healing site[c] | 3 | 4 | 2 | 3 | 5 | 3 | 4 | 4 |
| Small, single/few, poor healing site[c] | 2 | 3 | 3 | 2 | 2 | 1–2 | 5 | 7 |
| Large, single, poor healing site[c] | 3 | 2–3 | 5 | 4 | 5 | 1 | 6 | 7 |
| Facial | 4 | 7 | 2 | 2 | 4[d] | 3 | 4 | 7 |
| Digital | 3 | 7 | 3 | 5 | 2[d] | 3 | 3 | 3 |
| Perianal | 6 | 6 | 6 | 6 | 1[e] | 7 | 2–3 | 6 |
| Penile | 3 | 3 | 3 | 5 | 4[d] | 3 | 2–3 | 3 |

5-FU, 5-fluorouracil; PDT, photodynamic therapy; 1, probably treatment of choice; 2, generally good choice; 3, generally fair choice; 4, reasonable but not usually required; 5, generally poor choice; 6, probably should not be used; 7, insufficient evidence available. The suggested scoring of the treatments listed takes into account the evidence for benefit, ease of application or time required for the procedure, wound healing, cosmetic result, and current availability/costs of the method or facilities required. Evidence for interventions based on single studies or purely anecdotal cases is not included.

[a]Does not have a product license for Bowen's disease.

[b]Depends on site.

[c]Refers to the clinician's perceived potential for good or poor healing at the affected site.

[d]Consider micrographic surgery for tissue sparing or if poorly defined/recurrent.

[e]Wide excision recommended.

Topical imiquimod may be used off-label for Bowen's disease for larger lesions or difficult/poor healing sites[11] – SOR B. However, it is costly and the optimum regimen has yet to be determined.[11]

One prospective study suggests a superiority of curettage and electrodesiccation over cryotherapy in treating Bowen's disease, especially for lesions on the lower leg.[12] Curettage was associated with a significantly shorter healing time, less pain, fewer complications, and a lower recurrence rate when compared with cryotherapy.[12]

### Clinical Types and Locations

*Common type*

The edge of the patch is clearly demarcated but often irregular or scalloped, and the surface has a white or yellowy scale. Several lesions may appear close together or widely scattered. The morphological changes may be similar to those of a small psoriatic plaque (see Figures 9.22 and 9.23). Bowen's disease is often found on the fingers and hands related to exposure to human papillomavirus (HPV) (**Figure 9.24**).

*Hyperkeratotic*

The surface may be heaped up into a horn or a thick plaque (see Figure 9.23). Scale may be lost in the center.

### Bowen's Disease of the Glans Penis and of the Vulva and Perineum

Bowen's disease of the glans penis (erythroplasia of Queyrat) has a red velvety appearance (**Figure 9.25**). It should be differentiated from Zoon's (plasma cell) balanitis, psoriasis, lichen planus, scabies, and sexually transmitted infections. A shave biopsy is needed before cryosurgery to exclude progression to invasive malignancy. Bowen's

disease of the vulva, penis, and perineum (**Figure 9.26**) is still often referred to as bowenoid papulosis, but the official nomenclature is grade 3 vulval and penile intraepithelial

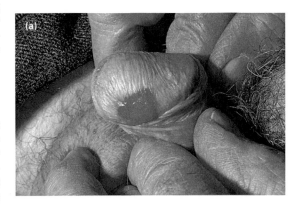

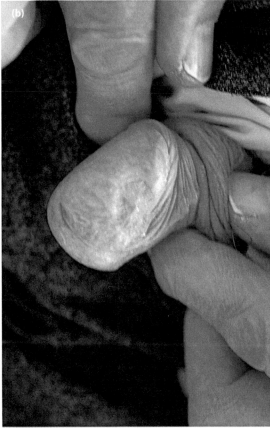

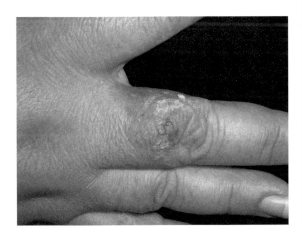

*Figure 9.24* Bowen's disease on the finger. The biopsy demonstrated human papillomavirus as the source of this squamous cell carcinoma in situ. (Courtesy of Richard Usatine, MD.)

*Figure 9. 25* (a) Bowen's disease of the glans penis (erythroplasia of Queyrat). (b) After treatment with one 30-s freeze–thaw cycle. No recurrence was seen up to 6 years later.

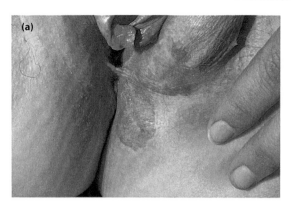
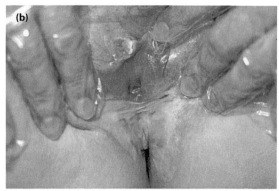

*Figure 9. 26* (a) Pigmented Bowen's disease of the vulva and perineum. (b) After cryosurgery with a single 30-s freeze–thaw cycle. The normal stretching of skin shows that no inelastic scar tissue has appeared, although hypopigmentation is obvious.

neoplasia (VIN and PIN). These lesions are strongly associated with HPV type-16 infection. Small papules (usually multiple and sometimes pigmented) appear on cutaneous and mucosal surfaces, and may resemble simple warts, seborrheic keratoses, or melanocytic nevi. Areas of erythema and erosion may also develop. There is a risk of progression to invasive malignancy. Biopsy will confirm clinical suspicions and help to exclude other dermatoses, including extramammary Paget's disease.

### Management of Bowen's Disease

Several methods give satisfactory cure rates. The most suitable will depend on the size and site of the plaque and the general condition of the patient. A biopsy should always be taken to establish the nature of the lesion and to exclude underlying squamous cell carcinoma.

Treatment options include the following:

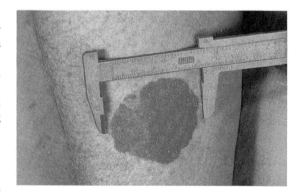

*Figure 9.27* Bowen's disease of the lower leg. Use of cryosurgery on this large lesion of the leg would likely result in delayed healing. Photodynamic therapy is an alternate mode of management in lesions of the lower limb. (Courtesy of Richard Usatine, MD.)

- For small thinner lesions, and particularly where the diagnosis is in doubt, curettage and electrosurgery are appropriate.
- For small thicker lesions, excision may be the best option.
- Topical therapy with 5-FU 5% cream or imiquimod 5% cream may be used.
- PDT is very useful for larger lesions, particularly on the lower limb (**Figure 9.27**).
- Cryosurgery: the spray technique is considered to be better than the cotton-wool bud technique (**Figure 9.28**). For Bowen's disease of the skin (not genitalia), a single 20- to 30-second spray after the icefield has been established is required, and at least 2 mm of healthy tissue should be included to ensure treatment of the complete lesion. Larger, more established lesions can be divided into overlapping circles using a skin marker and each circle treated with a

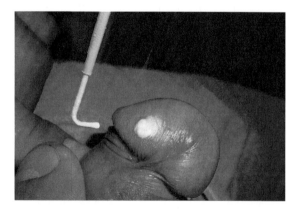

*Figure 9.28* (a) Bowen's papulosis (biopsy proven) of the glans penis being treated with cryosurgery and a bent tip spray. (Courtesy of Richard Usatine, MD.)

single 20-second freeze–thaw cycle (**Figure 9.29**). However, if there is concern about delayed healing (eg over the tibia), subsequent circles can be treated after a gap of a few weeks. Alternately, larger lesions, other than on the leg, may be treated using a single 20- to 30-second freeze using the spiral or paint-spray technique, ensuring at least a 2 mm clear margin of treatment. Markedly hyperkeratotic lesions do not respond well to cryosurgery alone, and should be "debulked" with curettage before cryosurgery.

For Bowen's disease of the genitalia, there are no studies comparing cure rates for different treatments or looking at

optimal freezing times with cryosurgery. A 15- to 20-second freeze–thaw cycle is recommended. Healing is usually rapid, giving excellent results in both functional and cosmetic terms (see Figures 9.25, 9.26, and 9.28).

Bowen's disease is often seen on the lower leg in older age groups, with a female preponderance, and not uncommonly with some features of underlying venous stasis. Aggressive cryosurgery can easily lead to ulceration and delayed healing (see Figures 9.23 and 9.27). There is only a small risk of malignant transformation, so careful judgment must be exercised when deciding whom and how to treat. A study by Ahmed et al. in 2000 highlighted this problem on the lower limb.[12] They compared cryosurgery

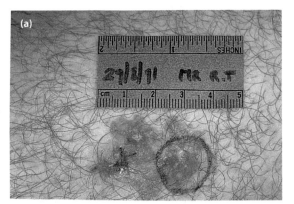
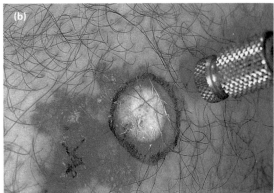
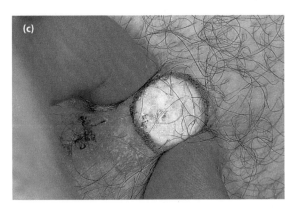
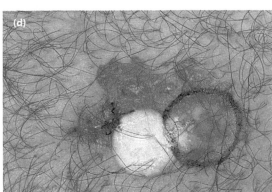
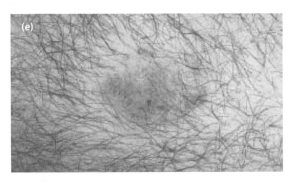

*Figure 9.29* Bowen's disease: (a) before cryosurgery; (b) during cryosurgery; (c) during cryosurgery – the icefield is palpated to ensure that the full skin thickness is uniformly frozen; (d) during cryosurgery; (e) after treatment by cryosurgery. This demonstrates how overlapping fields of freezing are used (see Chapter 2).

*Table 9.2* Comparison of Cryotherapy with Curettage in the Treatment of Bowen's Disease: a Prospective Study[12]

| | Cryosurgery (36 patients) | Curettage (44 patients) |
|---|---|---|
| | 2 × FTCs of 5–10 s | Cautery for hemostasis |
| Median healing time | 46 days | 35 days |
| Lesions taking >90 days to heal | 12 | 6 |
| Infections requiring antibiotics | 4 | 2 |
| Recurrences within 24 months | 13 | 4 |
| Average healing time for lesions | 90 days for 23 lesions | 39 days for 36 lesions on lower leg |

FTC, freeze–thaw cycle.

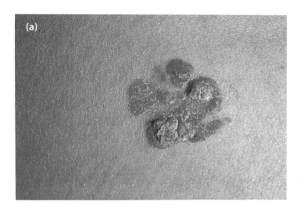

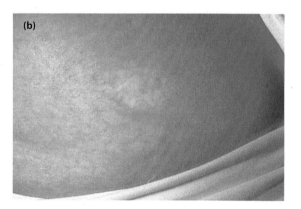

*Figure 9.30* **Bowen's disease: an irregularly hyperkeratotic patch: (a) before cryosurgery; (b) good results after cryosurgery. The patient was pleased with the treatment and outcome.**

with electrodesiccation and curettage for patients with Bowen's disease (most cases were on the lower leg, below the knee). A third of the patients treated with cryosurgery had lesions that took over 90 days to heal. Also the patients treated with cryosurgery had more infections of the healing site and a higher recurrence rate. The details are given in Table 9.2. However, Bowen's disease can be treated with cryosurgery on other areas of the skin with excellent cosmetic results, high patient satisfaction and reasonable cure rates (**Figure 9.30**).

With any premalignant disease, high cure rates must be weighed against side effects. No one will thank the physician who guarantees a cure at the expense of a slowly healing, painful ulcer. It is therefore justifiable to introduce a modicum of conservatism into this treatment. However, the dysplastic cells of Bowen's disease may extend down the appendiceal epithelium of hair follicles, where they are protected from superficial freezing. Recurrence is then common if the freeze is not aggressive because the cells migrate back to the surface, with new areas of Bowen's disease appearing in the middle of a previously treated site.

The evidence for the management of Bowen's disease was published in the guidelines by the British Association of Dermatologists.[11] They emphasized the difficulty of comparing studies because widely varying treatment regimens were used.

- They graded the use of cryotherapy for Bowen's disease as SOR B.
- They cited recurrence rates in the order of 5–10% provided that adequate cryosurgery is used (eg liquid nitrogen cryotherapy, using a single freeze–thaw cycle of 30 s, two freeze–thaw cycles of 20 s with a thaw period, or up to three single treatments of 20 s at intervals of several weeks).[11,13–15]
- In an RCT of PDT versus cryotherapy, cryosurgery produced 100% clearance in 20 patients with one to three treatments of liquid nitrogen, using

one freeze–thaw cycle of 20 s on each occasion (50% success after a single treatment). Ulceration was observed after cryotherapy in 25% of lesions. There were two (10%) recurrences after cryotherapy in the 1-year follow-up period. A single treatment of PDT was significantly more effective than cryotherapy.[15]

- Cryotherapy appears to have a good success rate with adequate treatment (recurrences <10% at 12 months) but healing may be slow for broad lesions and discomfort may limit treatment of multiple lesions. Curettage and PDT both have higher success rates and less discomfort overall, but are more time-consuming and/or expensive to perform.[11]
- Curettage followed by cryotherapy has also been used, but reports are anecdotal and it is impossible to determine the relative contribution of the two treatments or whether the combination is better than either alone.[11]

Treatment schedules for premalignant lesions are summarized in Table 9.3.

*Table 9.3* Recommendations for Treating Premalignant Conditions[a] (Using Liquid Nitrogen with an Open Spray Technique)

| Premalignant and malignant | Freeze time (s)[b] | Freeze–thaw cycles | Halo diameter (mm) |
|---|---|---|---|
| Actinic keratosis | 5–10 | 1 | 1 |
| Actinic cheilitis | 5–10 | 1–2 | 0 |
| Bowen's disease (genitalia) | 15–20 | 1 | 2 |
| Bowen's disease (skin) | 20–30 | 1–2 | 2 |

[a]Cryosurgery is a preferred treatment based on good evidence for actinic keratoses. It is also preferred for actinic cheilitis. Treatments for actinic keratoses and actinic cheilitis may be followed by topical treatments for better field treatment. Cryosurgery for Bowen's disease (squamous cell carcinoma *in situ*) is one option among many choices including surgery, electrodesiccation, and curettage based on the lesion, location, and patient preference.

[b]Freeze times: includes a range of times based on the variable sizes and locations of lesions. Smaller lesions on thinner more delicate skin should receive treatments at the lower end of the range. Patients receiving treatments of 20 s or more should be offered local anesthetic first. All times are based on the available studies and author experience.

## REFERENCES

1. Bonerandi JJ, Beauvillain C, Caquant L, et al. Guidelines for the diagnosis and treatment of cutaneous squamous cell carcinoma and precursor lesions. J Eur Acad Dermatol Venereol 2011;25(suppl 5):1-51.
2. Anwar J, Wrone DA, Kimyai-Asadi A, Alam M. The development of actinic keratosis into invasive squamous cell carcinoma: evidence and evolving classification schemes. Clin Dermatol 2004;22:189–96.
3. Criscione VD, Weinstock MA, Naylor MF, Luque C, Eide MJ, Bingham SF. Actinic keratoses: Natural history and risk of malignant transformation in the Veterans Affairs Topical Tretinoin Chemoprevention Trial. Cancer 2009;115:2523–30.
4. de Berker D, McGregor JM, Hughes BR. Guidelines for the management of actinic keratoses. Br J Dermatol 2007;156:222–30.
5. Smith SR, Morhenn VB, Piacquadio DJ. Bilateral comparison of the efficacy and tolerability of 3% diclofenac sodium gel and 5% 5-fluorouracil cream in the treatment of actinic keratoses of the face and scalp. J Drugs Dermatol 2006;5:156–9.
6. Hadley G, Derry S, Moore RA. Imiquimod for actinic keratosis: systematic review and meta-analysis. J Invest Dermatol 2006;126:1251–5.
7. Lebwohl M, Dinehart S, Whiting D, et al. Imiquimod 5% cream for the treatment of actinic keratosis: results from two phase III, randomized, double-blind, parallel group, vehicle-controlled trials. J Am Acad Dermatol 2004;50:714–21.
8. Siller G, Gebauer K, Welburn P, Katsamas J, Ogbourne SM. PEP005 (ingenol mebutate) gel, a novel agent for the treatment of actinic keratosis: results of a randomized, double-blind, vehicle-controlled, multicentre, phase IIa study. Australas J Dermatol 2009;50:16–22.
9. Zouboulis CC, Rohrs H. [Cryosurgical treatment of actinic keratoses and evidence-based review.] Hautarzt 2005;56:353–8.
10. Thai KE, Fergin P, Freeman M, et al. A prospective study of the use of cryosurgery for the treatment of actinic keratoses. Int J Dermatol 2004;43:687-692.
11. Cox NH, Eedy DJ, Morton CA. Guidelines for management of Bowen's disease: 2006 update. Br J Dermatol 2007;156:11–21.
12. Ahmed I, Berth-Jones J, Charles-Holmes S, O'Callaghan CJ, Ilchyshyn A. Comparison of cryotherapy with curettage in the treatment of Bowen's disease: a prospective study. Br J Dermatol 2000;143:759–66.
13. Cox NH, Dyson P. Wound healing on the lower leg after radiotherapy or cryotherapy of Bowen's disease and other malignant skin lesions. Br J Dermatol 1995;133:60–5.
14. Holt PJ. Cryotherapy for skin cancer: results over a 5-year period using liquid nitrogen spray cryosurgery. Br J Dermatol 1988;119:231–40.
15. Morton CA, Whitehurst C, Moseley H, McColl JH, Moore JV, Mackie RM. Comparison of photodynamic therapy with cryotherapy in the treatment of Bowen's disease. Br J Dermatol 1996;135:766–71.

# 10 Malignant lesions

With appropriate selection of patients and tumors, adequate equipment, and proper techniques, cryosurgery is an excellent therapeutic modality for the treatment of skin malignancies. Indeed, it may be the treatment of choice for some skin cancers and a good alternative in other settings. Cryosurgery is included as a treatment modality in the guidelines for non-melanoma skin cancer produced by organizations including the American Academy of Dermatology, the British Association of Dermatologists, and the Cancer Council of Australia.[1-4] As with other established techniques such as excisional surgery, electrosurgery and curettage, radiotherapy, and Mohs' surgery, cryosurgery has its own special advantages and limitations.

## PRINCIPLES OF TREATMENT

When treating skin cancers with cryosurgery the goal is destruction of the lesion at the first treatment. To accomplish this, the tumor must be frozen to a sufficient depth and with adequate peripheral margins so that no focus of malignancy remains untreated (**Figure 10.1**).

Most failures in cryosurgical treatment of skin cancers are due to the following:

- Poor tumor selection
- Poor technique.

Liquid nitrogen, with its temperature of −196°C, is the most reliable refrigerant for consistent cell destruction and is the only cryogen that we recommend for the treatment of skin cancers.

The important concepts involved have been discussed in the early chapters of this book. Tumors have unpredictable growth beneath the skin, often spreading laterally further than the surface changes would indicate. In contrast, the dermal ice produced by surface application of liquid nitrogen has a smaller diameter than suggested by the surface freeze. Bearing in mind the relationship between lateral freeze and depth of freeze, it is possible to predict approximately the size of the icefield required to treat a particular tumor. Just as the surgical margin would be 3–4 mm for most small-to-medium basal cell carcinomas (BCCs), so the icefield for such lesions should be 3–5 mm beyond the clinical margin to account for the fact that the edge of the ice ball is less cold. To achieve an adequate depth of cryogenically induced necrosis for most tumors, one should carry out a double 30-second freeze–thaw cycle, with a minimum 2-minute thaw period between each freeze.

Mallon demonstrated that BCCs below the head and neck respond equally well to a single 30-s freeze–thaw cycle.[5]

The recommended tissue temperature for tumor freezing is below −40°C. Previously this could be measured only with thermocouples inserted into the skin, but now it can be measured using the Cry-Ac TrackerCam technology from Brymill. This involves an infrared temperature sensor on the front of the cryospray unit. The light on the skin turns green when the temperature drops below 0°C and red when the temperature drops below whatever setting has been preset on the Cry-Ac TrackerCam (see Figure 3.8, Chapter 3). This allows for non-invasive temperature monitoring of the treatment for malignant skin lesions. Moreover, the clinician can film the procedure while monitoring the temperature and freeze times.

### Note on Preferred Aperture Tips for Cryosurgery

Although the bent spray tips are great for treating benign lesions with gentle liquid nitrogen spray velocities, they should be avoided when treating skin cancers. Preferred tips include the C- or-B aperture tips or a straight needle-type tip (see Figure 3.11). These tips allow sufficient flow for rapid freezing and low temperatures.

## TUMOR SELECTION

Several factors influence the decision to consider cryosurgical treatment, rather than other modalities, for a malignant lesion. For BCCs, these include the size of the lesion, and its site and histopathology but equally important are the experience of the operator and the available facilities. Squamous cell carcinoma (SCC) *in situ* and small SCCs may also be treated with cryosurgery (**Figure 10.2**). There is more controversy over the use of cryosurgery for SCCs because inadequate treatment leaves a small chance of metastatic spread of the tumor. Despite the general rule that cryosurgery should be restricted to the treatment of low-risk tumors there are circumstances in which it has a place in the management of large or recurrent tumors and those in special sites, but great experience is needed for this type of work.[6]

Cryosurgery is usually not the treatment of choice for the following:

- Tumors >2 cm diameter
- Recurrent tumors
- Tumors in areas of high risk for recurrence
- Tumors on lower limbs, where healing is poor

- Sclerosing BCCs
- Infiltrating and micronodular BCCs
- Most invasive SCCs (especially if there is perineural invasion)
- All melanomas
- All Merkel's cell carcinomas.

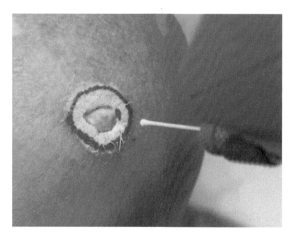

*Figure 10.1* Cryosurgery of a superficial basal cell carcinoma (BCC) on the shoulder using open spray of liquid nitrogen through a straight tip on a cryogun. A single 30-s freeze was performed. (Courtesy of Richard Usatine, MD.)

## PATIENT SELECTION

Having taken into account the features of the tumor that might make it more or less suitable for cryosurgery, it is also important to look at factors for individual patients that may favor this approach to treatment. The patient's age and state of health are important. Cryosurgery may be particularly suited to patients who are considered at poor risk for surgery and anesthesia or individuals not suitable for other forms of treatment. The ease with which a patient can attend for treatment may also be relevant, because one can treat elderly housebound patients by cryosurgery in their own homes or in a nursing home setting. Patients with dementia are more likely to tolerate cryosurgery rather than excisional surgery (**Figure 10.3**).

### Patient Information

In contrast to benign lesions, which only require short freeze times and no anesthesia, BCCs often require local anesthesia and a double 30-s freeze–thaw cycle.[5] The end result is usually excellent, but the inflammatory reaction of the malignancy and the surrounding tissues is considerable and complete healing may take several weeks.

Before treatment, it is most important to provide informed consent including a thorough explanation of all the possible side effects (see Box 6.1). This should include the swelling, which may not appear until the next day, the degree of pain, and the subsequent care of the treated area. The advice is best reinforced by an information sheet, which

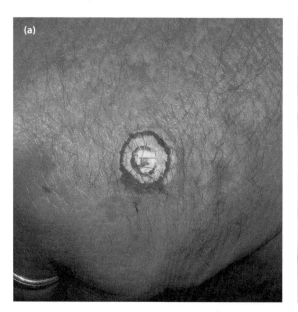

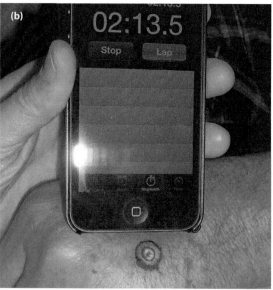

*Figure 10.2* (a) Squamous cell carcinoma in situ on the hand after cryosurgery applied with cryospray for a 30 s single freeze–thaw cycle. (b) Note that the thaw time is over 2 min and there is still some freezing at the center of the lesion. (Courtesy of Richard Usatine, MD.)

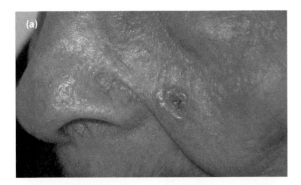

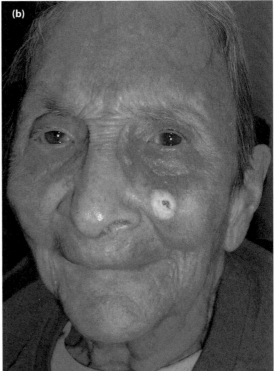

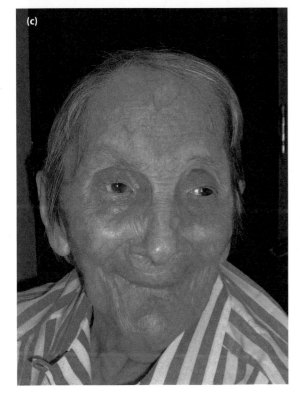

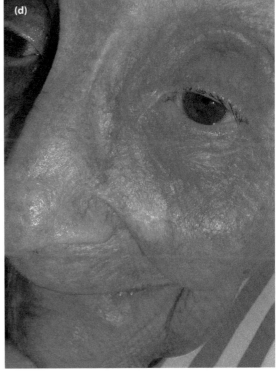

*Figure 10.3* (a) Basal cell carcinoma on the cheek of a 94-year-old woman with Alzheimer's disease. The patient was non-verbal and unable to understand her diagnosis or the treatment options. Her family chose cryosurgery for the treatment. The patient's head had to be held for the injection of local anesthetic. However, she did remain still for the cryosurgery which did not hurt. A double 30-s freeze–thaw cycle was used. (b) 7 months later at a follow-up visit there was no evidence of recurrence clinically and the patient was happy. (c, d) Close-up of the healed area showed some hypopigmentation and slight scarring. This was very acceptable to the family. (Courtesy of Richard Usatine, MD.)

the patient and relatives can read at their leisure (Box 10.1). Treatment of facial lesions may produce sufficient edema to close the eye, and this is seen most notably in the morning after lying recumbent overnight. It may help if patients sleep with their heads raised for a few days after a periocular lesion has been treated.

---

*Box 10.1* What to Expect After Cryosurgery of Skin Cancer

- After cryosurgery, the treated area will swell and may weep fluid. Gauze dressing is recommended for the first few days to absorb this fluid.
- If your skin cancer is on the face (especially if close to the eye) sleep with your head raised for a few days to minimize swelling around your eyes.
- The wound will form a hard, dry, black adherent crust after 10–14 days. It may be anything from a week to a month or more before it separates to leave a pink appearance. It may take months before your skin color returns and the final result may be lighter or darker than the original color.
- There should be relatively little pain after the procedure but acetaminophen every 4–6 hours can be taken if required. Severe pain or swelling may indicate the presence of secondary infection, in which case a course of antibiotics may be prescribed by your doctor.
- If any problems arise in connection with your cryosurgery, please contact your doctor.

---

### Tumor Histopathology

Although it is safe to "undertreat" a benign skin lesion, the degree of freeze given to a malignant lesion is crucial. It is therefore wise to take a pretreatment biopsy. A shave biopsy with local anesthesia is usually adequate. The results of the biopsy may help to determine the cryosurgical technique required or dissuade the clinician from using cryosurgery at all if, for example, the biopsy reveals an infiltrative BCC. Nodular BCCs or small, well-differentiated SCCs require a double 30-s freeze–thaw cycle whereas superficial BCCs may require no more than a single 30-s freeze–thaw cycle. If a biopsy has been performed, it is wise to wait at least 2 weeks until the inflammation settles, and any suture has been removed, before cryosurgery because otherwise prolonged bleeding can occur during the thaw phase.

### Clinical Varieties

There are three main types of BCC:

1. Nodular BCCs (**Figure 10.4**) are raised, with translucent pearly borders. Small telangiectatic vessels may appear on the surface. They may be ulcerated centrally, giving rise to the typical "rodent ulcer"

(**Figure 10.5**). These are the most common form of BCCs and may be pigmented. Some variants are micronodular and these are more difficult to eradicate.

2. Superficial BCCs (**Figure 10.6**) start as flat, red, slightly scaly patches, which spread and become more scaly. They may have a "whipcord" edge or "thready" border (**Figure 10.7**). They generally occur on the trunk. Spotty pigmentation may also occur in this type of BCC. Some appear to be multicentric.

3. Sclerosing (morpheaform) BCCs appear as waxy, indurated plaques. The borders are indistinct (**Figure 10.8**). These are the least common form of BCCs but the most aggressive biologically. Some may infiltrate widely even around nerves. We do not recommend using cryosurgery for this form of BCC.

Although these descriptions account for most BCCs, their appearance can vary widely and may imitate benign lesions such as seborrheic keratoses. For this reason it is always best to have a histologic diagnosis before initiating cryosurgical treatment. Any non-healing ulcer or new pearly papule in a sun-exposed area is suspicious for skin cancer and needs evaluation.

One of the best methods of evaluation before a biopsy is the use of a dermatoscope. Dermascopic evaluation can increase the sensitivity and specificity of diagnosis before the biopsy. It can also help direct the biopsy to the most clinically suspicious area (see Appendix C).

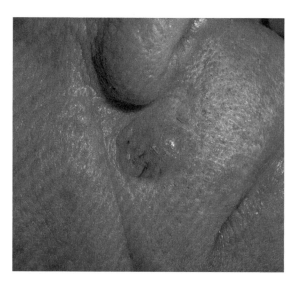

*Figure 10.4* **Typical pearly nodular BCC on the face. The proximity to the nasal ala and the nasolabial fold and lip would make this a challenging BCC to treat with cryosurgery. (Courtesy of Richard Usatine, MD.)**

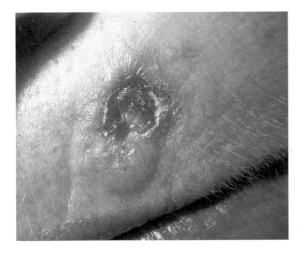

*Figure 10.5* Nodular BCC with ulceration on the upper lip. This relatively large nodular BCC is very close to the upper lip and cryosurgery could lead to tenting of the upper lip with an unappealing cosmetic result. (Courtesy of Richard Usatine, MD.)

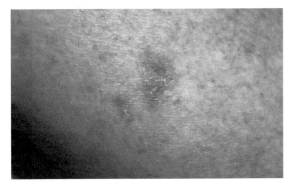

*Figure 10.6* Superficial BCC on the arm of a 60-year-old woman. (Courtesy of Richard Usatine, MD.)

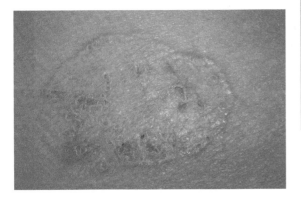

*Figure 10.7* Large superficial BCC on the back with a "thready border" or "whipcord" edge appearance.

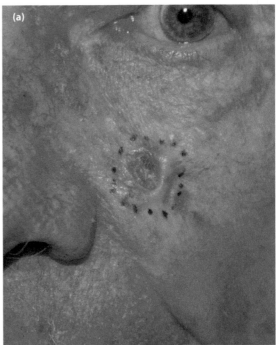

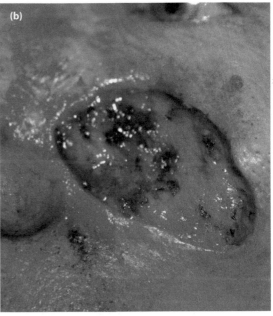

*Figure 10.8* (a) Sclerosing BCC that required many steps of Mohs' surgery for clear margins. Cryosurgery would most likely have resulted in recurrence as the tumor spread further than 5 mm around the visible margin. (b) Defect before closure. (Courtesy of Ryan O'Quinn, MD.)

## CRYOSURGERY FOR BCCs

Superficial BCCs of the type often seen on the trunk or extremities of elderly patients (see Figures 10.6 and 10.7), small lesions of the basal cell nevus syndrome (**Figure 10.9**), and small lesions on X-ray-damaged skin may be treated with a single freeze–thaw cycle. Swelling and morbidity will be less than after the double freeze–thaw cycle that is needed to eradicate solid, cystic, or ulcerated rodent ulcers.

Physicians embarking on cancer cryosurgery may consider starting by treating superficial BCCs that might otherwise be treated by electrodesiccation and curettage (**Figure 10.10**). Until greater skill has been acquired, it is

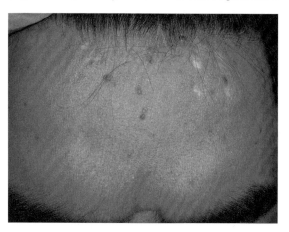

*Figure 10.9* Nevoid BCCs: this 29-year-old man with basal cell nevus syndrome has over 30 small BCCs on his face that appear similar to pigmented nevi. Treatment options include cryosurgery, electrodesiccation and curettage (ED&C) surgery, and oral vismodegib. The atrophic hypopigmented scars are from aggressive ED&C treatments in the past. (Courtesy of Richard Usatine, MD.)

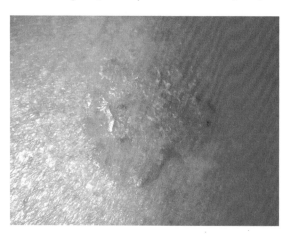

*Figure 10.10* Superficial BCC) on the back with a thready border and some spotty brown pigmentation. Although this superficial BCC is rather large at 2 cm in diameter, cryosurgery with a 30-s single freeze–thaw cycle is an acceptable alternative.

best to avoid the sites that have higher recurrence rates (eg the inner canthus, nasolabial folds, and periauricular lesions). For experienced cryosurgeons, the ear, eyelid, and cartilaginous parts of the nose are relatively good sites for cryosurgery because cartilage necrosis is not likely with routine methods[7–9] and connective tissue damage and distorting scars are rare.[10]

The tissue-sparing value of cryosurgery has special relevance for tumors on the eyelids. A reappraisal of cryosurgery of the eyelids by Buschmann emphasized the high cure rate and avoidance of ectropion.[11] Buschmann believes that cryosurgery should have an increasing role to play for tumors in this area, especially when probe delivery is used. He does state that sclerosing and thick tumors, and most tumors on the upper lid, are best managed by scalpel surgery (preferably with Mohs' surgery for margin control).[11]

In the case of a solid or cystic-type BCC, the lesion to be treated is first outlined with a marker pen, leaving a 3- to 5-mm clinically clear margin (**Figure 10.11**). If the margins are ill defined, surgery with pathologic confirmation of clear margins is a better option. The complete area to be treated is then infiltrated with 1% lidocaine and epinephrine. For a well-circumscribed malignancy, the liquid nitrogen is applied directly as a spray (**Figure 10.12**).

When a BCC has an irregular outline or is near to a structure that might need protection (eg the eye), adhesive putty can be used to circumscribe the lesion together with a 3- to 5-mm margin. Eye protection can also be performed with a tongue depressor, which can be wrapped with gauze for added protection (**Figure 10.13**). A double freeze–thaw cycle is then carried out to achieve subzero temperatures (preferably reaching less than −40°C). Each of the two freeze times is 30 s with a minimum intervening thaw time of 2 min.

If a superficial BCC larger than 2 cm in diameter is to be treated, it is best to use a circular or spray-paint technique (see Figure 5.8) to ensure adequate freeze across the total lesion. This may require longer freeze times to freeze the whole lesion as the 30-s freeze time is based on the spot-freeze technique.

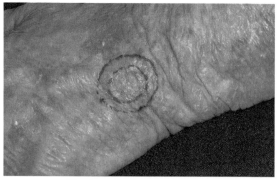

*Figure 10.11* Superficial BCC marked before cryosurgery. It is safe to perform cryosurgery on the dorsum of the hand for a superficial BCC. (Courtesy of Richard Usatine, MD.)

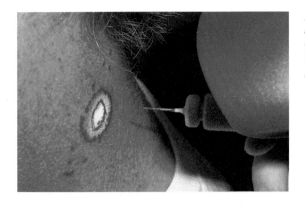

*Figure 10.12* Cryosurgery of a BCC on the neck. An elliptical excision that could be performed was drawn on the skin to show the patient the available options during informed consent. The patient chose cryosurgery over the elliptical excision. (Courtesy of Richard Usatine, MD.)

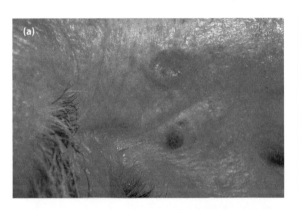

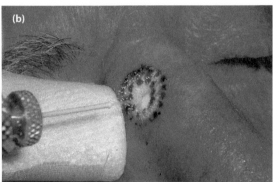

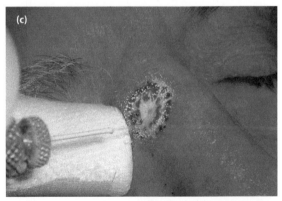

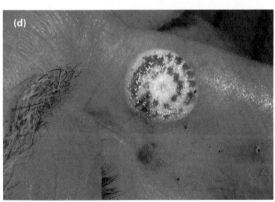

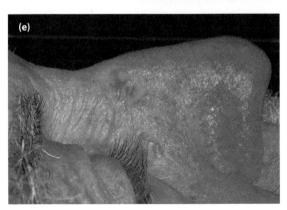

*Figure 10.13* Cryosurgery of a nodular BCC on the nose of a 66-year-old man. The patient had had previous skin cancers removed by surgery, ED&C, and cryosurgery. Cryosurgery was his preference even when Mohs' surgery was presented as an alternative covered by his insurance. (a) The original nodular BCC before shave biopsy. (b) Cryosurgery with a gauze-wrapped tongue depressor to protect the eye. Note the marked borders and 4-mm halo diameter. The green light indicates a surface temperature of less than 0°C. (c) Cryosurgery continues with an open cryosurgery and a red light indicating a surface temperature of less than −20°C. (d) Final ice ball after a double 30-s freeze–thaw cycle. (e) The healed cryosurgical site 2 months later. (Courtesy of Richard Usatine, MD.)

## One or Two Freeze–Thaw Cycles

In a study of cryosurgery for BCCs, a 95.3% cure rate was achieved in the treatment of facial BCCs with a double freeze–thaw cycle.[5] This compared with a cure rate of only 79.4% when facial lesions were treated with a single freeze–thaw cycle. Treatment of superficial truncal BCCs with a single freeze–thaw cycle achieved a cure rate of 95.5%. One 30-s freeze–thaw cycle to superficial truncal BCCs appears adequate.[5] Note that nodular truncal BCCs were not studied so that it might be best to use a double 30-s freeze–thaw cycle for these thicker tumors.

## Curettage and Cryosurgery

There are a number of studies that combine curettage with cryosurgery in the treatment of BCCs.[12] Curettage is performed to debulk the BCC before the cryosurgery. As there are no comparison studies of cryosurgery with and without curettage, we do not know if curettage increases the cure rate.

In one study of curettage with cryosurgery, 69 patients with 100 non-facial tumors, ≤2 cm in diameter, consisting of superficial BCC, small nodular BCC with papillary dermal invasion, squamous cell carcinoma (SCC) *in situ*, and SCC with papillary dermal invasion were prospectively treated with this technique. They were then evaluated at 1- and 5-year intervals. No tumor recurred after 1 year of follow-up, and one recurrence occurred within the 5-year interval, for a 99% recurrence-free endpoint.[13]

The step-by-step details for curettage and cryosurgery in this one study (for tumors not on the face and only superficial BCC) are:[13]

- Margins of 4 mm are drawn around the visible border of the tumor.
- Local anesthesia is achieved with 1% lidocaine and epinephrine.
- Curettage is performed in multiple directions with a sharp, disposable curette until all friable tumor tissue and epidermis have been removed from within the marked margins, leaving a clinically uniform, normal-appearing, normal-feeling dermal base.
- Hemostasis is achieved with 20% aluminum chloride.
- The entire curetted field is treated broadly using a continuous liquid nitrogen spray, aimed at a distance of 5 mm, using a paint-brush method.

One freeze–thaw cycle with freeze times of 10–20 s is performed.[13]

In a study of 136 consecutive patients with 171 difficult-to-treat BCCs (secondary to size >1 cm, location, nature, or patient condition), tumors were treated by the mixed technique of curettage followed by liquid nitrogen application. After an average follow-up of 5.2 years (6 months to 9.1 years), a cure rate of 91.8% was achieved. These lesions were curetted with small-diameter curettes (2–4 mm) and Monsel's solution was applied to achieve hemostasis. Liquid nitrogen was delivered by spray technique or cryoprobes and a double freeze–thaw cycle was used.[6]

In a study by Thissen et al., curettage using a sharp curette was performed under local anesthesia (lidocaine 1% without epinephrine). Initially a large curette was used to debulk the tumor mass. Finally, a small curette was used to remove the remainder of the BCC around the borders. Monsel's solution was used to perform hemostasis. A liquid nitrogen spray was used to freeze the tissue. A double 20-s freeze–thaw cycle was used.[14]

Our step-by-step recommendations for curettage and cryosurgery of BCCs (based on the literature and author experience) are as follows:

- Local anesthesia with 1% lidocaine and epinephrine.
- Curettage is performed in multiple directions with a sharp, disposable curette until all friable tumor tissue has been removed (**Figure 10.14**).
- Hemostasis is achieved with aluminum chloride.
- Mark 3- to 5-mm margins around the curetted area with a marking pen.
- The entire curetted field with margins is treated using a continuous liquid nitrogen spray (if the tumor is large, the spray can be performed with the paint-brush technique or in four separate quadrants).
- One or two freeze–thaw cycles with freeze times of 20–30 s are performed depending on the depth and location of the BCC. Facial and thicker tumors should receive a double freeze–thaw cycle with longer freeze times.

Kuflik often prefers curettage before cryosurgery to debulk the tumor and aid in delineation of the lesion.[15] If there are any questions about the border of the BCC, curettage can provide additional information before drawing the cryosurgery margins. This also reduces the amount of tissue that must be frozen and may speed healing by reducing the volume of tissue that must slough.[15] As preliminary curettage has not been shown to alter the cure rate, its use is a matter of personal preference. Debulking the tumor can also be performed with a shave followed by curettage (Figure 10.14).

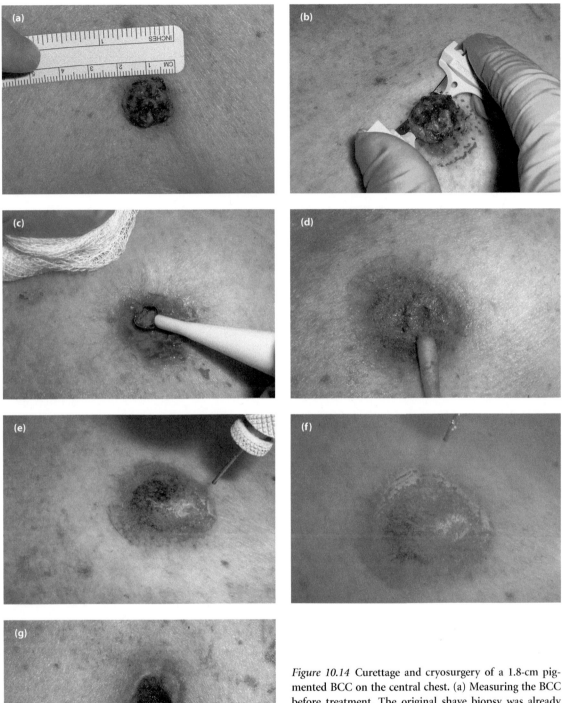

*Figure 10.14* Curettage and cryosurgery of a 1.8-cm pigmented BCC on the central chest. (a) Measuring the BCC before treatment. The original shave biopsy was already healed. (b) Shave excision to debulk the BCC before cryosurgery. (c) Curettage to further debulk the BCC. (d) Aluminum chloride applied for hemostasis before cryosurgery. (e) Cryosurgery performed with an open-spray spot-freeze technique to the first quadrant. (f) Second quadrant treated with spot-freeze technique. (g) Eschar 1 week after cryosurgery. (Courtesy of Richard Usatine, MD.)

*Clinical examples*

1. Treatment of BCC with monitoring of temperature (**Figure 10.15**):
   - A marker pen is used to draw a 3- to 5-mm margin around a BCC on the arm. Local anesthetic with 1% lidocaine and epinephrine is administered and the temperature is monitored with the Cry-Ac TrackerCam.
   - Small nodulocystic BCC on the arm before shave biopsy. As the shave biopsy removed all the visible tumor, no curettage was needed before cryosurgery.

   - The ice ball is starting to form as the tracker light has turned green to indicate that the surface temperature has dropped below 0°C.
   - The tracker light has turned red as the surface temperature has dropped below −40°C and the full ice ball has been established. The freeze time was 30 s.
   - The ice ball can be palpated to feel the depth and breadth of the freeze.
   - Thawing of the lesion with prominent erythema at the margins. The center takes longer to thaw as expected, but once it did so a second freeze–thaw cycle of 30 s was performed.

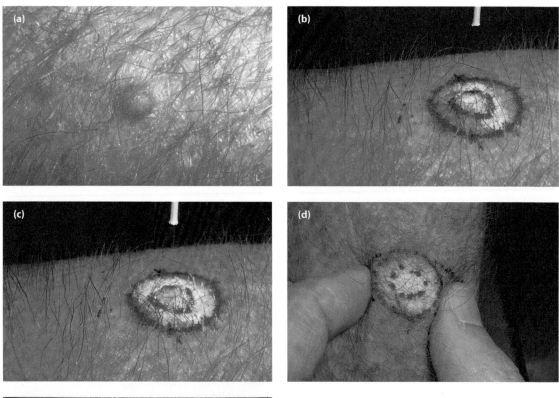

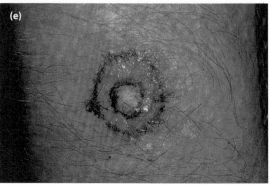

*Figure 10.15* (a) Cystic BCC on the arm proven by biopsy. (b) Cryosurgery of this cystic BCC with the green light indicating a surface temperature of <0°C. (c) Cryosurgery continues with red light indicating a surface temperature of less than −40°C. (d) Note how the freeze ball is like a frozen disk that can be palpated between the fingers. (e) Thawing of freeze ball with some remaining ice at the center. (Courtesy of Richard Usatine, MD.)

2. Comparison of cryosurgery and electrosurgery on the face (**Figure 10.16**):
   - Two small nodular BCCs, one on the nose and the other on the cheek (see arrows), were diagnosed with shave biopsies.
   - Cryosurgery is performed and the ice ball starts to thaw after the first of two 30–s freeze–thaw cycles.
   - Electrodesiccation and curettage (three cycles) were performed on the small BCC on the nose with visible char. The cryosurgery site on the cheek shows erythema.

- Healed treatment areas 9 months later. Note the hypopigmentation and minor skin atrophy in both locations. Years later there were no recurrences and the patient was happy with the results. When asked, he preferred the cryosurgery overall and stated that it was less painful during the healing process.

## SQUAMOUS CELL CARCINOMA
Risk factors for the development of SCC include sun exposure, immunosuppression, aging, certain chronic skin diseases, human papillomaviruses, and burns.

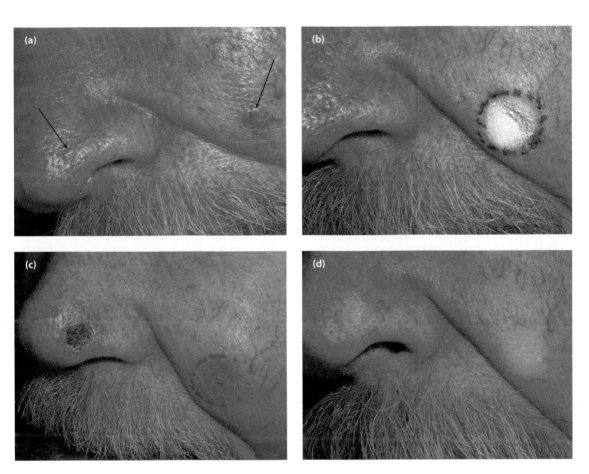

*Figure 10.16* Comparison of cryosurgery and electrosurgery on the face of a 55-year-old man: (a) two small nodular BCCs, one on the nose and the other on the cheek (see arrows). (b) Cryosurgery ice ball visible and starting to thaw after the first of two 30-s freeze–thaw cycles. (c) Electrodesiccation and curettage (three cycles) were performed on the nose with visible char remaining. The cryosurgery site on the cheek shows erythema. (d) Healed treatment areas 9 months later. Note the hypopigmentation and minor skin atrophy in both locations. (Courtesy of Richard Usatine, MD.)

## Clinical Varieties

The most common sites for SCCs of the skin are the face, neck, back of the hand, and forearm (**Figure 10.17**). SCCs usually present as a firm, indurated, expanding nodule, not uncommonly associated with pre-existing actinic keratoses. The lower lip and ear are common sites with higher rates of metastases and therefore less favorable sites for cryosurgery.

SCCs grow laterally and vertically, and may metastasize to local draining lymph nodes or distant sites. Well-differentiated tumors have a keratinous surface, which may range from a thin soft keratin layer to a rock-hard horn. The less well-differentiated tumors may have no keratin and appear as wet, red masses simulating granulation tissue or a pyogenic granuloma. Not infrequently, SCCs become ulcerated.

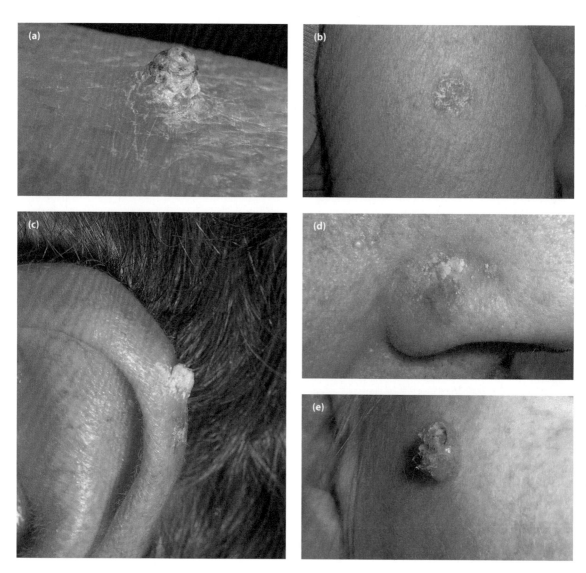

*Figure 10.17* (a) Cutaneous horn on the arm of a 65-year-old woman, which grew rapidly over 6 months. Biopsy revealed a squamous cell carcinoma (SCC) of the keratoacanthoma type. The base of this lesion could easily be treated with a double freeze–thaw cycle using liquid nitrogen by cryospray. (b) This SCC on the arm of a woman could be frozen using a double freeze–thaw cycle with liquid nitrogen by cryospray. (c) This small keratosis on the pinna turned out to be a well-differentiated SCC arising in an actinic keratosis. This is one SCC that could be treated safely with cryosurgery. (d) This small SCC on the nasal ala could be treated by cryosurgery. There is some risk of notching and Mohs' surgery would be preferred if available. (e) This SCC of the keratoacanthoma type was diagnosed with a shave biopsy. Treatment options include elliptical excision, cryosurgery, and electrodesiccation and curettage. (Courtesy of Richard Usatine, MD.)

The clinical signs of SCCs in the early stages are less clear-cut than those of BCCs. Therefore diagnosis before cryosurgery of an SCC is essential. In fact, SCCs on sun-exposed skin are one end of a spectrum of disease that starts with actinic keratosis, progresses to SCCs *in situ* (Bowen's disease), and then becomes invasive SCCs. See Chapter 9 for treatment recommendations of actinic keratoses and Bowen's disease.

### Cryosurgery for SCCs

The treatment of even well-differentiated SCCs requires a double 30-s freeze–thaw cycle with a 5-mm lateral clear margin to avoid failure or recurrence (**Figures 10.18, 10.19 and 10.20**).[16] SCCs are more likely to invade underlying

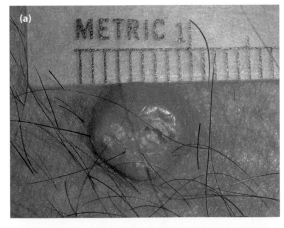

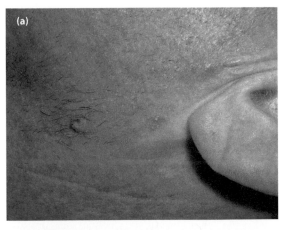

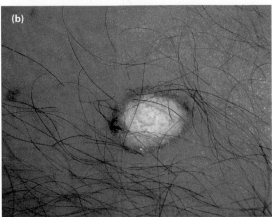

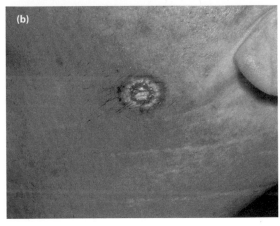

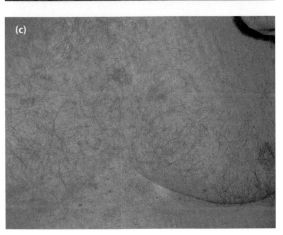

*Figure 10.18* (a) Well-differentiated squamous cell carcinoma on the face of a 51-year-old man. (b) Note how the lesion was circled with a surgical marker and the 5-mm halo margin marked before cryosurgery. (Courtesy of Richard Usatine, MD.)

*Figure 10.19* (a) A keratoacanthoma grew quickly on the center of the chest of this 72-year-old man. (b) The patient chose to have cryosurgery when the biopsy results were known. Cryosurgery was performed with a double 30-s freeze–thaw cycle. (c) Eight years later there has been no recurrence. (Courtesy of Richard Usatine, MD.)

tissue such as cartilage and, if aggressive cryosurgery is used on the ear, a permanent structural defect may occur. Even though good cure rates can be obtained, cryosurgery is probably best avoided for treatment of SCCs on the ear (**Figure 10.21**).

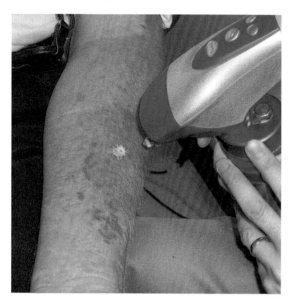

*Figure 10.20* Cryosurgery of a well-differentiated SCC on the arm. This SCC was treated with a double freeze–thaw cycle and 5-mm margins. (Courtesy of Richard Usatine, MD.)

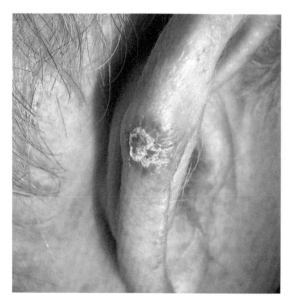

*Figure 10.21* SCC of the ear. This is best treated by Mohs' surgery and not cryosurgery. (Courtesy of Richard Usatine, MD.)

In a study by Kuflik and Gage, 52 SCCs were treated with a 5-year cure rate of 96.1%.[16] Liquid nitrogen was used to achieve tissue temperature in the cancer range of −40 to −60°C (measured with thermocouples). When there was difficulty in determining the extent of the lesion, preliminary curettage was used. The frozen tissue was allowed to thaw without assistance, then the cycle was repeated. The goal was to include an adequate margin of normal tissue in the frozen area of at least 3–5 mm. The total freeze time, depending on the size and thickness of the cancer, ranged from 40 s to 90 s for a 1- to 1.5-cm lesion. The highest recurrence rate for all SCCs (and BCCs) over 20 years was for tumors of the ear.[16]

In a later study by Kuflik, using the same cryosurgical technique, he treated 132 SCCs between 1990 and 1996, and there were no recurrences at the 5-year follow-up.[15] Preliminary curettage was carried out for most lesions except for thin SCCs. The open-spray technique was generally employed because of its versatility and speed. The author preferred the open-spray technique because the cryosurgical unit can be maneuvered easily to enable treatment of irregularly shaped lesions and those on curved areas. In a study by Holt, 1 of 34 (2.9%) SCCs recurred after treatment with cryosurgery.[17]

Excisional surgery or use of Mohs' surgery may be the treatment of choice for SCCs on the ear but, in some circumstances, and if the needed surgical skills are not available, cryosurgery is an option that should be considered. Nordin published a series of consecutive auricular non-melanoma skin cancers treated by curettage and cryosurgery.[18] His article gives a detailed description of the issues surrounding this treatment modality. Some 71 patients with 81 tumors were available for follow-up of at least 5 years and there was only one recurrence.[18] The cosmetic results were good or acceptable in most patients. Although we are not recommending this as a first-line modality, it is helpful to know that cryosurgery may be a backup when other approaches are not available.

## LENTIGO MALIGNA

Lentigo maligna is a term for melanoma *in situ* occurring on sun-exposed areas, especially on the face of elderly individuals. The original lesion usually begins by resembling a simple lentigo or large freckle, often on the temple or cheek. After many years, there is a gradual increase in size, with greater variation of pigment and irregularity of the margin, but the lesion remains macular (**Figure 10.22**). If biopsied at this stage, the lesion will show neoplastic melanocytes confined to the epidermis. Precancerous melanosis, preinvasive lentigo maligna, and Hutchinson's melanotic freckle are all synonyms. If left untreated, the lesion will continue to expand laterally. After a variable period of time, an invasive phase may develop and the lesion is then termed a "lentigo maligna melanoma" (LMM) (**Figure 10.23**). At this stage, the tumor has developed the capacity for metastatic spread.

The invasive growth phase may be accompanied by increased or decreased pigmentation and nodular change.

Taking an appropriate biopsy from suspected lentigo maligna is not straightforward. Sampling one area may miss invasive changes in another part of the lesion. The National Comprehensive Cancer Network (NCCN) Melanoma Guidelines state: "For lentigo maligna, melanoma *in situ*, a broad shave biopsy may help to optimize diagnostic sampling."[19] But if invasion is strongly suspected the NCCN recommends an excisional biopsy with 1- to 3-mm margins. This may be challenging in certain sites such as the eyelid or ear. However, the risks of incomplete sampling

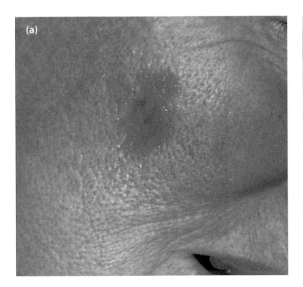
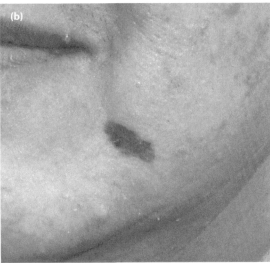

*Figure 10.22* (a) This large lentigo maligna is best treated by surgical excision for a high cure rate. Alternate treatments include topical imiquimod and cryosurgery. (With permission from Usatine RP, Moy RL, Tobinick EL, Siegel DM. Skin Surgery: A practical guide. St. Louis, MO: Mosby; 1998.) (b) This smaller lentigo maligna is best treated by surgical excision for the highest cure rates. If surgery is not an option, the smaller size and the patient's lighter skin color make cryosurgery an alternative to consider. (Courtesy of Richard Usatine, MD.)

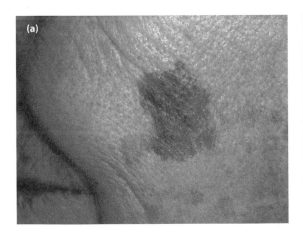
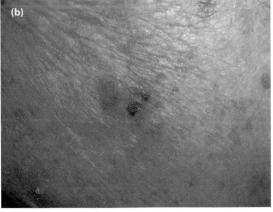

*Figure 10.23* (a) This large lentigo maligna melanoma should be surgically excised for the highest cure rate. Cryosurgery is not a good option. (Courtesy of the Skin Cancer Foundation; for more information visit www.skincancer.org). (b) Lentigo maligna melanoma on the face of a 65-year-old woman with sun-damaged skin was found to have a depth of 0.35 mm by broad shave biopsy. The patient was sent for Mohs' surgery. (Courtesy of Richard Usatine, MD.)

were highlighted in one study, which revealed that 16% of lesions that were diagnosed as lentigno maligna based on incisional biopsy were found to have foci of invasion (LMM) on complete excision.[20]

Once a diagnosis of lentigo maligna has been established many clinicians believe that surgical excision is the standard of care treatment[21] but other treatment options include cryosurgery, topical imiquimod, and laser and radiation therapy. The indistinct border and field change effect mean that no treatment is always effective. The site, patient's age, and state of health will influence the decision about the best approach.

With the increasing availability of Mohs' surgery and plastic surgical techniques involving staged excisions, cryosurgery is not the treatment of choice for most cases of lentigo maligna. However, dermatologists have been using cryosurgery to treat lentigo maligna for over 40 years.[22,23] Dawber and Wilkinson published a series of 14 cases of lentigo maligna treated with aggressive liquid nitrogen spray in 1979. They reported that the results were curative in all 14 patients.[22] Zacarian treated 20 patients with lentigo maligna with cryosurgery between the years 1973 and 1980. The tumors ranged in size from 1.0 cm to 7.0 cm (average size, 2.7 cm). The recurrence rate for all 20 patients was 10% (mean average period for follow-up evaluation was 42.6 months).[23]

In a study published in 2007, 18 patients with clinical and histopathologic diagnosis of lentigo maligna were treated with cryosurgery because the lesion posed a surgical challenge or the patient was not a good surgical candidate.[24] They were treated with two freeze–thaw cycles of liquid nitrogen under local anesthesia in a single sitting. The diameter of the lentigo maligna lesions varied from 2.5 cm to 6 cm (mean 4 cm). The frozen area was extended 1 cm beyond the visible borders of the lesion. Two freezing cycles of 1 min each were separated by a thaw cycle of at least 2 min. Lesions larger than 2 cm² were divided into smaller segments for freezing. The lesions resolved clinically in all cases, with no recurrence or metastasis detected during a mean follow-up of 75.5 months. Note that this was a particularly aggressive treatment with longer freeze times of 1 min and larger freeze margins of 1 cm. Healing times were 4–6 weeks for small lesions and 2–3 months for larger ones.[24]

## Cryosurgery for Lentigo Maligna (in Special Circumstances as Discussed Above) (Figure 10.24)

1. Biopsy for diagnosis is essential (Figure 10.24b). Informed consent that cryosurgery may not be the treatment of choice for lentigo maligna when surgical excision can be performed. Higher cure rates are more likely achieved with surgical excision.[21,24]
2. Local anesthesia with injectable lidocaine. The lesion should be outlined with a 3- to 5-mm lateral clear margin to ensure adequate depth and lateral spread of cryosurgery and cell death (Figure 10.24b).
3. Double 30-s freeze–thaw cycle. The exact freezing method will depend on the site and size of the lesion, but the method used should ensure an even depth of freeze across the total lesion (Figure 10.24d,e).
4. Adequate follow-up or supervision of patient progress.

## Palliation

Excisional surgery is the treatment of choice for invasive malignant melanoma. However, cryosurgery can play a palliative role in some cases (**Figure 10.25**). Kuflik published an article on cryosurgery for palliation in 1985.[25]

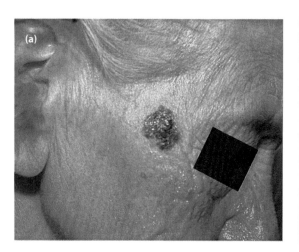
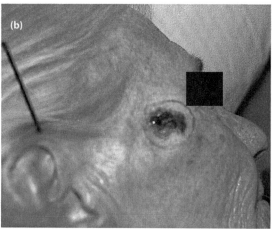

*Figure 10.24* (a) Lentigo maligna in an 80-year-old woman. (b) The lesion has been outlined with a clear margin and an edge biopsy has been carried out.

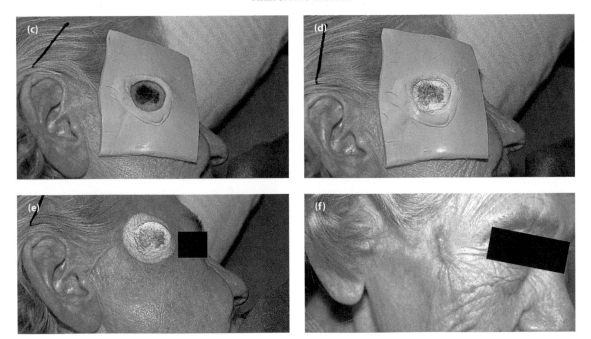

*Figure 10.24* (c) Protective adhesive putty in place. (d) After a 30-s cryofreeze. (e) The adhesive putty has been removed shortly after a second 30-s freeze (note the extent of the icefield). (f) At 6 months' review (the hypertrophic scar subsequently flattened spontaneously).

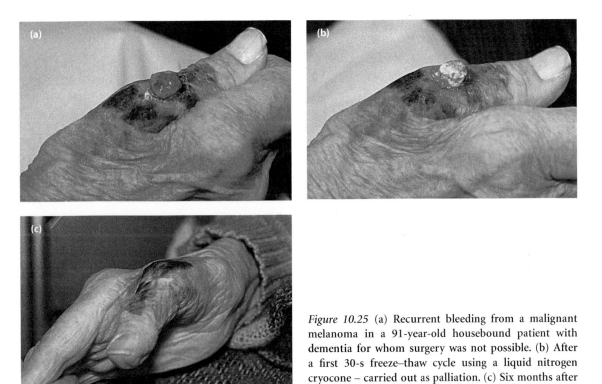

*Figure 10.25* (a) Recurrent bleeding from a malignant melanoma in a 91-year-old housebound patient with dementia for whom surgery was not possible. (b) After a first 30-s freeze–thaw cycle using a liquid nitrogen cryocone – carried out as palliation. (c) Six months after cryosurgery: good healing and symptom free.

113

He described how cryosurgery was a useful therapy for some "incurable" malignant skin lesions.[25] **Figure 10.26** illustrates the use of cryosurgery for a proven LMM in an 89-year-old patient who refused any other surgical intervention.

### RECURRENCE AND FOLLOW-UP FOR SKIN CANCER

These are the reasons to follow up patients after cryosurgery:

- Care of the wound
- Reassurance about the final cosmetic outcome
- Looking for signs of recurrence
- Monitoring for the development of new skin cancers.

Studies have shown that most recurrences following cryosurgery are detected 12–18 months after treatment.[17] However, as in any treatment for skin cancer, recurrences can occur more than 10 years after the treatment has been performed.[26]

A meta-analysis of studies of non-melanoma skin cancers showed a 3-year cumulative risk of a subsequent BCC after an index BCC of 44%, and the 3-year cumulative risk of a subsequent SCC after an index SCC of 18%.[27] These risks are at least a 10-fold increase in incidence compared with the rate in a comparable general population.[27] Therefore, routine follow-up of patients with skin cancers every 6–12 months is sensible in order to pick up early malignancies or recurrences.

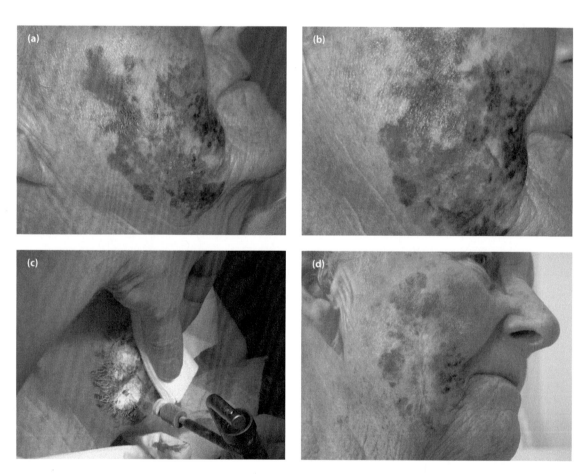

*Figure 10.26* (a) Lentigo maligna melanoma on the right cheek. A mentally alert but fairly immobile 89-year-old woman with two histologically proven lentigo maligna melanoma nodules at the sites marked and lentigo maligna at a more peripheral site. The patient refused any other surgical intervention. Cryosurgery was discussed, offered, and accepted. (b) Both nodular lentigo maligna melanomas have been outlined with 5-mm margins. (c) Both melanoma lesions are treated with a double 30-s freeze–thaw cycle under local anesthesia. (d) A considerable weepy reaction was experienced after cryosurgery, but both wounds healed well at 4 months. Thinner lentigo maligna areas were subsequently treated with a double 20-s freeze–thaw cycle to prevent further progression of the lesion, clearing pigmentation and improving cosmesis. The patient continued to do well, with no signs of recurrence at the 2-year follow-up.

## SUMMARY OF TREATMENT SCHEDULES

Treatment schedules for malignant lesions are summarized in Table 10.1.

*Table 10.1* Recommendations for Treating Malignant Conditions[1] (Using Liquid Nitrogen with an Open-Spray Technique)

| Type of lesion | Freeze time average (s)[a] | Freeze–thaw cycles | Halo diameter (mm) |
|---|---|---|---|
| Superficial BCC (not on face) | 15–30 | 1 | 3–5 |
| Nodular BCC (not on face) | 30 | 2 | 3–5 |
| BCC (face) | 30 | 2 | 3–5 |
| Keratoacanthoma | 30 | 2 | 4–5 |
| SCC *in situ* (Bowen's disease) | 30 | 2 | 4–5 |
| SCC | 30 | 2 | 4–5 |

[a]Cryosurgery for *in situ* and malignant conditions is only one treatment option and the others, including surgery, electrodesiccation and curettage, and Mohs' surgery, should be discussed with the patient. Cryosurgery should not be used for sclerosing or infiltrative BCC and any cancer with perineural invasion. BCC, basal cell carcinoma; SCC, squamous cell carcinoma.

## REFERENCES

1. Cancer Council Australia/Australian Cancer Network. Basal Cell Carcinoma, Squamous Cell Carcinoma (and Related Lesions) – A guide to clinical management in Australia. Sydney: Cancer Council Australia and Australian Cancer Network, 2008.

2. Motley R, Kersey P, Lawrence C. Multiprofessional guidelines for the management of the patient with primary cutaneous squamous cell carcinoma. Br J Dermatol 2002;146:18–25.

3. Drake LA, Ceilley RI, Cornelison RL, et al. Guidelines of care for basal cell carcinoma. The American Academy of Dermatology Committee on Guidelines of Care. J Am Acad Dermatol 1992;26:117–20.

4. Telfer NR, Colver GB, Morton CA. Guidelines for the management of basal cell carcinoma. Br J Dermatol 2008;159:35–48.

5. Mallon E, Dawber R. Cryosurgery in the treatment of basal cell carcinoma. Assessment of one and two freeze–thaw cycle schedules. Dermatol Surg 1996;22:854–8.

6. Jaramillo-Ayerbe F. Cryosurgery in difficult-to-treat basal cell carcinoma. Int J Dermatol 2000;39:223–9.

7. Nordin P, Larko O, Stenquist B. Five-year results of curettage–cryosurgery of selected large primary basal cell carcinomas on the nose: an alternative treatment in a geographical area underserved by Mohs' surgery. Br J Dermatol 1997;136:180–3.

8. Nordin P. Curettage-cryosurgery for non-melanoma skin cancer of the external ear: excellent 5-year results. Br J Dermatol 1999;140:291–3.

9. Burge SM, Shepherd JP, Dawber RP. Effect of freezing the helix and the rim or edge of the human and pig ear. J Dermatol Surg Oncol 1984;10:816–19.

10. Shepherd JP, Dawber RP. Wound healing and scarring after cryosurgery. Cryobiology 1984;21:157–69.

11. Buschmann W. A reappraisal of cryosurgery for eyelid basal cell carcinomas. Br J Ophthalmol 2002;86:453–7.

12. Kokoszka A, Scheinfeld N. Evidence-based review of the use of cryosurgery in treatment of basal cell carcinoma. Dermatol Surg 2003;29:566–71.

13. Peikert JM. Prospective trial of curettage and cryosurgery in the management of non-facial, superficial, and minimally invasive basal and squamous cell carcinoma. Int J Dermatol 2011;50:1135–8.

14. Thissen MR, Nieman FH, Ideler AH, Berretty PJ, Neumann HA. Cosmetic results of cryosurgery versus surgical excision for primary uncomplicated basal cell carcinomas of the head and neck. Dermatol Surg 2000;26:759–64.

15. Kuflik EG. Cryosurgery for skin cancer: 30-year experience and cure rates. Dermatol Surg 2004;30:297–300.

16. Kuflik EG, Gage AA. The five-year cure rate achieved by cryosurgery for skin cancer. J Am Acad Dermatol 1991;24:1002–4.

17. Holt PJ. Cryotherapy for skin cancer: results over a 5-year period using liquid nitrogen spray cryosurgery. Br J Dermatol 1988;119:231–40.

18. Nordin P, Stenquist B. Five-year results of curettage–cryosurgery for 100 consecutive auricular non-melanoma skin cancers. J Laryngol Otol 2002;116:893–8.

19. Coit DG, Andtbacka R, Bichakjian CK, et al. Melanoma. J Natl Compr Canc Netw 2009;7:250–75.

20. Hazan C, Dusza SW, Delgado R, Busam KJ, Halpern AC, Nehal KS. Staged excision for lentigo maligna and lentigo maligna melanoma: A retrospective analysis of 117 cases. J Am Acad Dermatol 2008;58:142–8.

21. Nadiminti H, Scope A, Marghoob AA, Busam K, Nehal KS. Use of reflectance confocal microscopy to monitor response of lentigo maligna to nonsurgical treatment. Dermatol Surg 2010;36:177-184.

22. Dawber RP, Wilkinson JD. Melanotic freckle of Hutchinson: treatment of macular and nodular phases with cryotherapy. Br J Dermatol 1979;101:47–9.

23. Zacarian SA. Cryosurgical treatment of lentigo maligna. Arch Dermatol 1982;118:89–92.

24. de Moraes AM, Pavarin LB, Herreros F, de Aguiar MF, Velho PE, de Souza EM. Cryosurgical treatment of lentigo maligna. J Dtsch Dermatol Ges 2007;5: 477–80.

25. Kuflik EG. Cryosurgery for palliation. J Dermatol Surg Oncol 1985;11:867–9.

26. Torre D. Cryosurgery of basal cell carcinoma. J Am Acad Dermatol 1986;15:917–29.

27. Marcil I, Stern RS. Risk of developing a subsequent nonmelanoma skin cancer in patients with a history of nonmelanoma skin cancer: a critical review of the literature and meta-analysis. Arch Dermatol 2000;136:1524-–30.

# 11  Side effects and complications

Cryosurgery is used so often that it would be easy to forget the importance of explaining, in detail, the benefits and risks to every patient. The clinician must not only be aware of all detrimental effects but should be able to quantify the relative risk of these occurrences for each patient according to his or her age, the anatomical site, and the biology of the lesion. Cryosurgery is a destructive tool and can produce surprising side effects after relatively non-aggressive treatment schedules.

Many of the changes, seen after freezing tissue, are inflammatory and probably important in the success of the treatment. In other words, morbidity and side effects cannot always be treated as separate entities in cryosurgery. Some unwanted effects are specific to the regimen employed and to the site, pathology, and size of the lesion and these have been described in other chapters. Box 11.1 lists the chief complications and side effects. We consider in more detail the more common and most important effects because it is imperative that anyone performing cryosurgery should be well versed in this area.

## DATA FROM RECENT STUDIES

In a prospective study, patients with untreated actinic keratoses >5 mm in diameter on the face and scalp were treated with cryosurgery.[1] Eligible lesions received a single freeze–thaw cycle with liquid nitrogen given via a spray device and were reviewed 3 months thereafter. The only treatment criteria were complete freezing of actinic keratoses with a 1-mm rim of normal skin. Some 90 adult patients from the community with 421 eligible actinic keratoses were treated.[1]

A total of 49 discrete local adverse events were recorded during the study that could be directly attributable to cryosurgery. The most common events were stinging, pain, or a burning sensation (52%), erythema (16%), and edema (10%). Other events included blistering, skin infection, crusting, itch, and peeling. The majority (74%) of adverse events were recorded as mild and almost all the moderate and severe events were recorded in the pain category. All events resolved within 1 week, with no long-term sequelae. There were no reported serious adverse events.[1]

In another study, 48 basal cell carcinomas (BCCs) were frozen with two cycles of 20 seconds using liquid nitrogen spray.[2] In nearly 90% of the cases (42 of 48 tumors), patients complained of moderate-to-severe swelling of the treated area, followed by long-lasting leakage of exudate from the defect. Secondary wound infections treated with systemic antibiotics were seen in three cases (6%).[2]

---

**Box 11.1** Side Effects and Complications in Cryosurgery

**Temporary**

Early onset – common, expected (especially longer freezes)
- Pain during the freezing, thawing, and healing
- Blister formation – sometimes hemorrhagic
- Intradermal hemorrhage
- Edema around treatment site
- Weeping of fluid (especially after treating cancer)

Early onset – less common
- Headache affecting forehead, temples, and scalp
- Syncope

Delayed onset – less common
- Postoperative infection
- Hemorrhage from the wound site
- Pyogenic granuloma
- Delayed healing after moderate freeze to thin sun-damaged scalp

**May be permanent**

Common
- Hypopigmentation (most common and most visible in persons of color)

Uncommon
- Milia
- Atrophic or depressed scar
- Hypertrophic scars
- Neuropathic pain at cryosurgery site

Very uncommon
- Nail dystrophy (when treating periungual warts or myxoid cysts)
- Tendon damage, especially on the fingers
- Ectropion and notching of eyelids
- Tenting or notching of the vermilion border of the lip, ear, or ala of nose
- Alopecia
- Neuroma accompanied by recurrence of mucocele on the lip
- Erosive pustular eruption on the scalp
- Trigger for vitiligo

---

Jaramillo-Ayerbe used a double freeze–thaw cycle of liquid nitrogen spray or cryoprobes for difficult-to-treat BCC.[3] During the procedure, no complications were documented. Pain was present in the first 12 hours after cryosurgery and lasted usually no longer than 48 hours; it was described as slight to moderate. Edema was also present and remarkable, especially in large periocular or centrofacial treated lesions, and persisted for 1–10 days. The surface of the wound exuded a bloody and watery discharge, which gradually subsided and was replaced by an adherent crust.

Between 5 and 9 weeks, complete re-epithelialization caused the crust to peel off. One patient bled on postoperative day 15, and this stopped when compression was applied for a couple of hours. Four patients developed a painful cellulitic and suppurative process on the wound which required oral antibiotic administration. One patient developed ala nasi cartilage necrosis, which required surgical reconstruction. The wounds healed with variable degrees of hypopigmentation, which in most cases repigmented in the long term. Some hypertrophy of scar tissue was commonly observed in the first few months and finally resolved after 1–2 years. Cryosurgical scars tended to retract, especially in tumors involving the lips, inferior lid, and infraorbital region. An initial ectropion was commonly seen, but partially resolved after several months so that none of the patients needed surgical correction. On the scalp, eyebrows, and eyelashes, irreversible alopecia of the cryo-treated area was invariable. Of 171 treated tumors, 14 (8.2%) recurred, yielding a cure rate of 91.8%.[3]

## PAIN

All patients feel some degree of discomfort when local anesthesia is not used but it varies from patient to patient. Longer freeze times may cause little discomfort in some individuals, whereas others (especially children) are upset by short freezes. Of course, the fear that young children may experience directly impacts their perception of pain. Even the shortest cotton-wool bud freezes give a perceptible "burning" sensation. Methods that cause rapid lowering of temperature and ice formation often produce discomfort within seconds. Pain during the thaw phase, particularly after "tumor dose" methods, may last for many minutes and may be profound. Certain anatomic sites are more likely to produce pain – particularly the fingers (pulp and periungual area), the helix and concha of the ear, the lips, the temples, and the scalp. Even though pain is usually transient, a throbbing sensation after freezing the digits may persist for 1–2 hours (**Figure 11.1**). This may be lessened by elevating the affected extremity above the level of the heart.

Headache is not uncommon when lesions on the forehead, temples, and scalp are frozen, and it may last from minutes to hours. The headache is not always near the site of freezing. This is likened to the headache some people get when eating ice cream.

The issue of pain raises the question of the need for local anesthesia. In general, single-freeze schedules used for benign or pre-neoplastic skin lesions will not require local anesthesia. Topical anesthetics such as EMLA (lidocaine and prilocaine) cream applied 1–2 hours before cryosurgery may minimize pain. Alternately, another topical

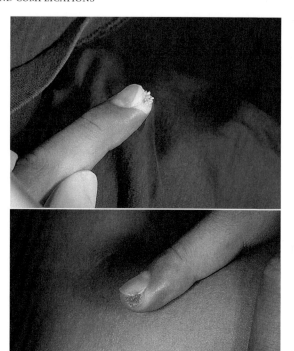

*Figure 11.1* "Over-zealous" cryosurgery of a periungual wart in a teenage boy resulted in severe throbbing pain of the finger and noticeable swelling of the distal digit. (Courtesy of Usatine R, Moy R, Tobinick E, Siegel D. Skin Surgery: A practical guide. St. Louis, MO: Mosby, 1998.)

anesthetic such as tetracaine may be used in advance of the cryosurgery. However, the best method to reduce pain during the longer freeze times used for treating malignancies is to inject lidocaine with or without epinephrine before initiating cryosurgery.

## BLISTER FORMATION

Blister formation can occur even with the short freeze times used to treat actinic keratoses and warts (**Figure 11.2**). If sufficient capillary and venular damage occurs then painless hemorrhagic bullae may develop within 12–24 hours. It is best to warn patients about this temporary side effect to avoid unnecessary phone calls and return office visits. The blisters may be left intact or punctured with a sterile needle when the blister is either large or uncomfortable. Whether or not the blisters are hemorrhagic, they will heal rapidly without scarring. Of course, if the blister is secondary to an aggressive cryosurgery of skin cancer and accompanied by deeper tissue necrosis, scarring can be expected (**Figure 11.3**).

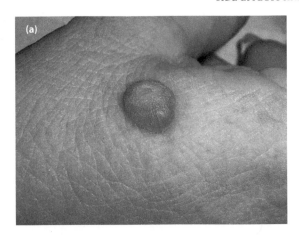

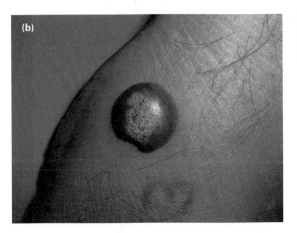

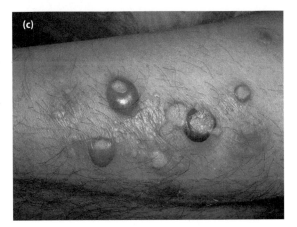

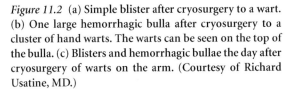

*Figure 11.2* (a) Simple blister after cryosurgery to a wart. (b) One large hemorrhagic bulla after cryosurgery to a cluster of hand warts. The warts can be seen on the top of the bulla. (c) Blisters and hemorrhagic bullae the day after cryosurgery of warts on the arm. (Courtesy of Richard Usatine, MD.)

## EDEMA

Some edema is seen with every patient as a result of the acute inflammation and "leaky" capillaries. The amount of edema is generally dose related but some people develop an idiosyncratic response even after short freeze schedules. The severest edema is typically seen after aggressive cryosurgery for skin cancer (**Figures 11.4 and 11.5**) in lax skin sites such as the eyelids (**Figure 11.6**), lips, labia minora (less commonly in the labia majora), and foreskin. When cryosurgery was used to treat BCCs with two 20-s freeze–thaw cycles, nearly 90% of the cases (42 of 48 tumors) resulted in moderate-to-severe swelling of the treated area.[2] Weeping of fluid may occur for days after the edema from the aggressive cryosurgical treatment of skin cancer.

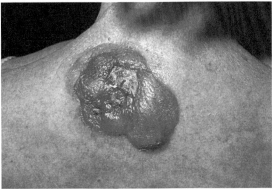

*Figure 11.3* Hemorrhagic blister and necrosis 3 days after aggressive treatment of a large basal cell carcinoma. This degree of inflammatory reaction may be minimized by clobetasol cream or a single dose of prednisolone 30 mg 2–3 hours before treatment.

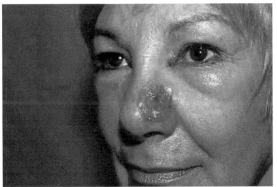

*Figure 11.4* Typical swelling reaction after satisfactory cryosurgery to a basal cell carcinoma on the nose. This healed well by 6 weeks.

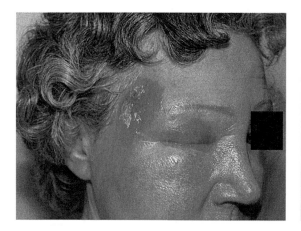

*Figure 11.5* Edema of the periorbital tissue may occur after aggressive freezing of lesions on the temple, as here, and the forehead.

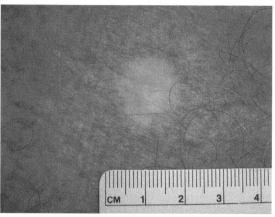

*Figure 11.7* Permanent hypopigmentation after a double freeze–thaw cycle using liquid nitrogen spray for a basal cell carcinoma on the chest. (Courtesy of Richard Usatine, MD.)

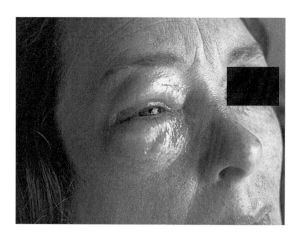

*Figure 11.6* Eyelid edema after treatment for xanthelasma. The lax tissues make them susceptible to these changes. Swelling began within 2 hours of treatment and remitted within 2 days.

## HYPOPIGMENTATION

Hypopigmentation is a common side effect of cryosurgery because melanocytes are more prone to cell death than keratinocytes. The longer freezes used for skin cancers are more likely to produce hypopigmentation (**Figures 11.7–11.9**). Although hypopigmentation is often permanent it can be temporary (**Figure 11.10**).

In one study of cryosurgery for BCCs, the wounds healed with variable degrees of hypopigmentation and in most cases the site repigmented in the long term.[2] Patients should always be cautioned about potential hypopigmentation and cryosurgery should be avoided or used carefully for patients with dark skin types.

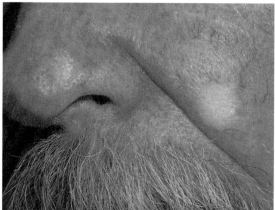

*Figure 11.8* Permanent hypopigmentation with some skin atrophy on the cheek after cryosurgery with double freeze–thaw cycle using liquid nitrogen spray for basal cell carcinoma (BCC). The atrophic hypopigmented scar on the nose was secondary to electrodesiccation and curettage of another BCC. Both treatments were performed on the same day so that the patient could compare the two methods. The patient preferred the cryosurgery and requested cryosurgery treatment for BCCs in the future. (Courtesy of Richard Usatine, MD.)

## HEMORRHAGE AND VASCULAR NECROSIS

Within 4–7 days of aggressive cryosurgery (mainly tumor schedules), it is not uncommon for the treated field to become cyanosed, with subsequent necrosis ("venous" gangrene) and subsequent sloughing (**Figures 11.11 and 11.12**).

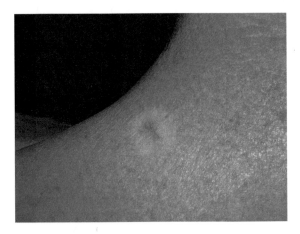

*Figure 11.9* Permanent hypopigmentation with slight skin atrophy after an aggressive double freeze–thaw cycle using liquid nitrogen spray for a basal cell carcinoma in an HIV-positive man. The patient was pleased with the result. (Courtesy of Richard Usatine, MD.)

This is probably due to delayed thrombosis of capillaries and venules, and may be an important and necessary part of tumor death and high cure rates (**Figures 11.13 and 11.14**).

Hemorrhage may occur with cryosurgery by several mechanisms. If a pedunculated or prominently papular lesion is manipulated during its solid ice phase, any ice cracks that appear may be associated with bleeding during the thaw – this is usually capillary/venous bleeding and is transient. If cryosurgery is preceded by biopsy or curettage (eg to "debulk" tumors) then postfreeze bleeding may last many minutes but is easily controlled by application of aluminum chloride solution or electrocoagulation. However, it is preferable to control the bleeding of biopsy or curettage with aluminum chloride (or Monsel's solution) before starting the cryosurgery.[2–4]

The least common and most dramatic form of hemorrhage is the delayed type which can occur up to 14 days after treatment. This may relate to a delayed necrotic phase after treatment of a tumor that had already invaded large arterioles. Bleeding of this type may be profuse and

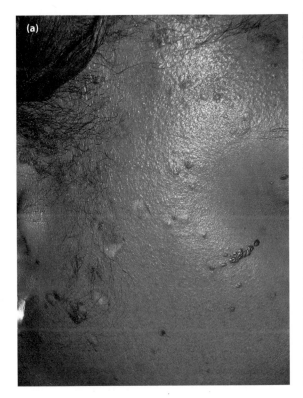

*Figure 11.10* (a) Temporary hypopigmentation that occurred on the face of a black woman after treatment of dermatosis papulosis nigra with a gentle cryospray. She was warned of this side effect and stated that she would prefer flat hypopigmentation, which she could cover with makeup, to the raised seborrheic keratoses on her face.

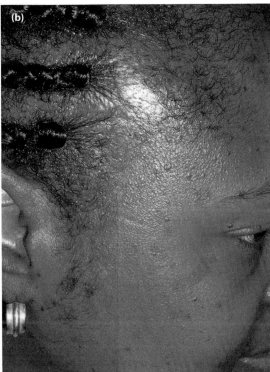

*Figure 11.10* (b) Hypopigmentation was only temporary and after a few additional treatments the patient was very pleased with the outcome. (Courtesy of Richard Usatine, MD.)

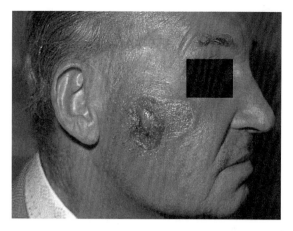

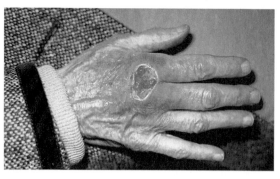

*Figure 11.14* Erosion after two freeze–thaw cycles of liquid nitrogen spray for squamous cell carcinoma on the dorsum of the hand. Such lesions heal without the need for grafting, mainly because undamaged dermal connective tissue in the wound promotes healing without contractile scarring.

*Figure 11.11* "Vascular" necrosis 6 days after double freeze–thaw cycle of a 2-cm diameter basal cell carcinoma. Healing tissue remains undamaged and promotes re-epithelialization.

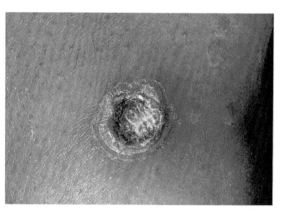

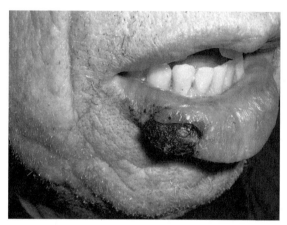

*Figure 11.12* Deep eschar formation after a hemorrhagic and necrotic phase, following the treatment of Bowen's disease below the knee.

*Figure 11.15* Bleeding complication after cryosurgery of a venous lake on the lip of a man taking coumadin. The venous lake was treated with liquid nitrogen using a cryoprobe applicator. Bleeding was not excessive but did produce an unsightly blood clot. (Courtesy of Richard Usatine, MD.)

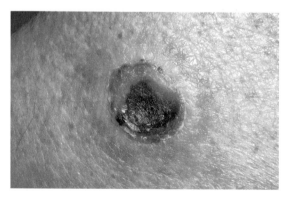

dangerous, requiring immediate pressure and early tying of the affected vessel. One patient bled from a deep vulvar artery 11 days after a single freeze–thaw cycle for multicentric pigmented Bowen's disease and required transfusion of 4 pints of blood. Patients on coumadin may be at higher risk (**Figure 11.15**).

### INHIBITION OF INFLAMMATORY COMPLICATIONS

Most of the complications described above are the results of various components of the acute or chronic inflammatory reactions caused by freezing. Many attempts have been made to minimize or avoid these effects without compromising cure rates. Some experts state that swelling

*Figure 11.13* Eschar 17 days after double 30-second freeze–thaw cycles of a basal cell carcinoma on the shoulder of an HIV-positive man. There was no pain or tenderness and the lesion healed well over time. The final result can be seen in Figure 11.9. (Courtesy of Richard Usatine, MD.)

and blister formation may be lessened by using topical clobetasol or oral prednisone (bolus-dose or short-term use). There are no data to support this for routine use.

## SENSORY IMPAIRMENT

Some degree of paresthesia, or less commonly anesthesia, is common after freezing. Indeed, the fact that cold can produce numbness has been known for many centuries. The analgesic effect of cryosurgery has proved effective in the palliative management of various inoperable tumors by direct application to the tumor, whereas cryoprobes have also been used to produce analgesia in patients with intractable pain by blocking peripheral nerve function. These studies have also shown that, although all transmission is blocked in the frozen nerve, full recovery occurs after a variable period (**Figure 11.16**).[5,6] This supports previous work directly freezing the sciatic nerve of rabbits with liquid nitrogen; in all cases, nerve conduction was completely interrupted, but, within 100 days, measurements confirmed full restoration of normal function. Thus, if a nerve trunk underlying a treated skin lesion is inadvertently damaged, complete recovery of distal sensory or motor function can be expected.

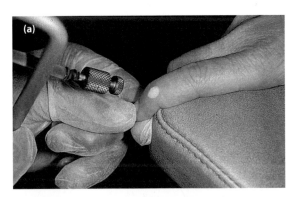

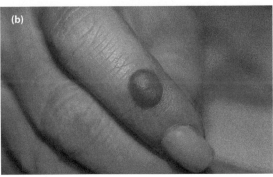

*Figure 11.16* (a),(b) "Over-zealous" cryosurgery of a finger wart resulted in a hemorrhagic blister and distal finger numbness for 4 months. (Courtesy of Usatine R, Moy R, Tobinick E, Siegel D. Skin Surgery: A practical guide. St. Louis, MO: Mosby, 1998.)

A study by Sonnex showed that appreciation of all three modalities of sensation tested (touch, pain, and cold) was initially reduced in all patients studied (**Figure 11.17**).[5] The recovery took up to 1.5 years for the longest freeze. Compared with control skin, all treated areas sampled within the first few weeks of cryosurgery were found to have an absence of axons in the upper dermis and a noticeable reduction in the deeper dermis. The longer the freeze time, the more pronounced were these changes. Even with the longest freeze time, however, Schwann cell and connective tissue pathways were present in normal numbers at all levels, with areas of Schwann cell proliferation. Apart from mild lymphocytic infiltration around a few of the neurovascular bundles, there was little evidence of inflammation and minimal fibroblastic activity. Dilation of occasional superficial blood vessels was the only vascular change detected. Biopsy specimens taken at later stages contained increasing numbers of axons at all levels.

Faber et al. carried out sensory testing by means of a graded bristle technique after treatment of 183 skin lesions in 169 patients.[6] Mild transient sensory loss was detected in 28% of treated lesions. This did not appear to be influenced by the freezing technique used or the type of wound healing, but was site dependent: the trunk and neck gave more prolonged impairment than the face, but sensory loss was not detected at all on the eyelid.[6] It is these effects that may be the basis of the successful use of cryosurgery to decrease pruritus in pruritus vulvae, pruritus ani, lichen sclerosus, prurigo nodularis, and lichen simplex chronicus.

## SKIN ATROPHY AND SCARRING

Skin atrophy and scarring are rare after therapeutic doses of cryosurgery for benign lesions (**Figure 11.18**). Cryosurgical regimens that involve severe and prolonged freezing of the skin for skin cancer are capable of producing skin atrophy and hypertrophic scarring (**Figures 11.18–11.20**).[7] Preservation of the fibrous network within the skin is typical after cryosurgery; this acts as a network around which cellular components regenerate. As a result, the cosmetic result is often excellent, although dermal thinning may be a feature in the long term. Fibroblasts appear to be less susceptible to damage by freezing than epidermal cells.

Cartilage necrosis is extremely rare after freezing (**Figure 11.21**), and good cosmetic results can be expected after cryosurgery of ear, eyelid, and nasal lesions. It should be remembered that the only consistent exception to this is cartilage already invaded by tumor. Even if tumor cure is achieved a cartilage defect may occur. This is more likely with squamous cell carcinoma than basal cell carcinoma (**Figure 11.22**).

Scarring includes the effects on adventitious glands of the skin and hair follicles. Follow-up histology after tumor treatments consistently reveals loss of sweat, sebaceous and apocrine gland structures; indeed, this has led to cryosurgery being used in some centers to treat hidradenitis

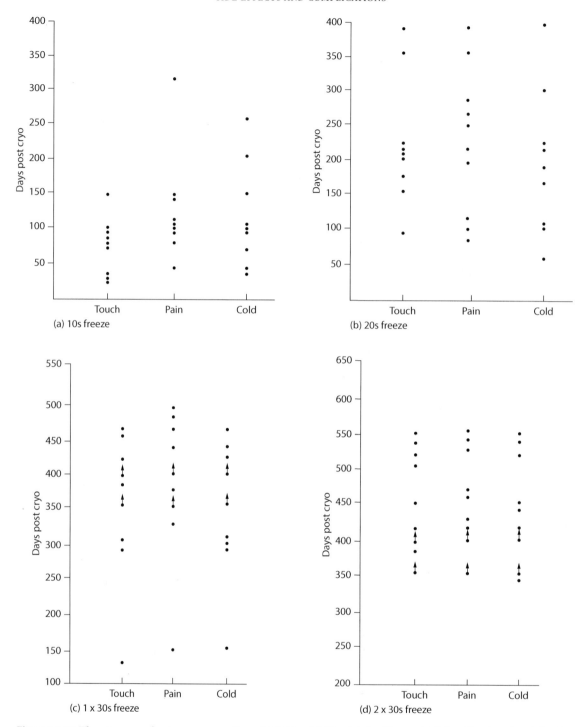

*Figure 11.17* The response of cutaneous sensation of (a) 10 s, (b) 20 s, (c) 1 × 30 s, and (d) 2 × 30 s duration (after ice formation). The individual results represent the time at which that modality of sensation returned to normal. (Courtesy of Sonnex TS, Jones RL, Weddell AG, Dawber RP. Long-term effects of cryosurgery on cutaneous sensation. Br Med J (Clin Res Ed) 1985;290:188–90.)

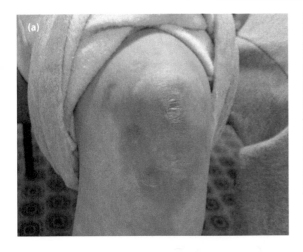

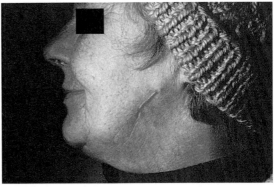

Figure 11.20 A linear hypertrophic scar 6 months after treatment of squamous cell carcinoma.

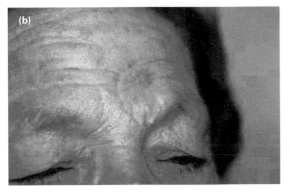

Figure 11.18 (a) Atrophic scarring from "over-zealous" cryosurgery to warts on the knee. (b) Atrophic hypopigmented scarring in a 69-year-old woman after aggressive cryosurgery for an infiltrative basal cell carcinoma of the forehead. The patient refused any other surgical intervention and was "happy" with the outcome.

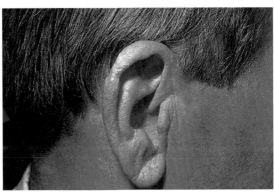

Figure 11.21 The ear 4 months after double freeze–thaw cycle therapy for basal cell carcinoma. Only slight skin atrophy has occurred, but there is no cartilage damage.

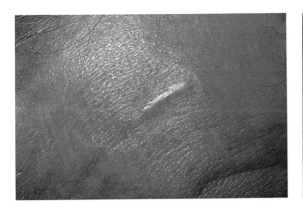

Figure 11.19 A linear hypertrophic scar 10 weeks after treatment (two freeze–thaw cycles) of a basal cell carcinoma; scarring of this type usually remits spontaneously within 6–9 months.

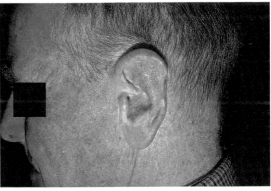

Figure 11.22 Ear cartilage loss 4 months after cryosurgery for squamous cell carcinoma that had invaded the cartilage.

suppurativa, various components of acne vulgaris, and axillary hyperhidrosis. Loss of the larger, normal, sebaceous pores after nasal and centrifacial skin treatments significantly alters the appearance of the skin and contributes greatly to the difficulty of cosmetically masking such blemishes (**Figure 11.23**).

The nose is particularly prone to visible scarring that can be cosmetically unappealing. For that reason, Mohs' surgery is considered the treatment of choice for skin cancers on the nose. **Figures 11.24 and 11.25** show two examples of nasal scarring including nasal rim "notching."

## ALOPECIA

Hair follicle damage after all but the shortest freeze times is so consistent (**Figure 11.26**) that cryosurgery of the scalp and beard area may be best reserved for the treatment of small lesions. Of course in men with male-pattern baldness, the use of cryosurgery is a very acceptable treatment of actinic keratoses on the bald scalp. Burge and Dawber

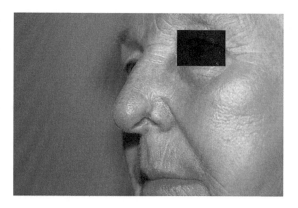

*Figure 11.25* Nasal rim "notching" 6 months after cryosurgery for squamous cell carcinoma.

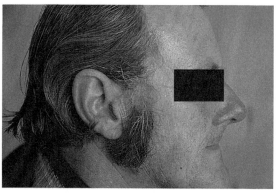

*Figure 11.26* Permanent hair follicle loss in the sideburn after a single 10-s freeze of a flat seborrheic keratosis.

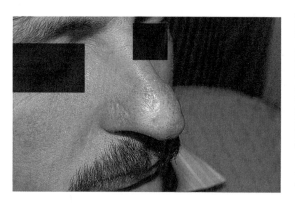

*Figure 11.23* Loss of pilosebaceous pores and slight hypopigmentation after focal treatment of early rhinophyma.

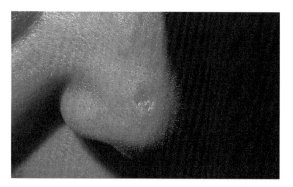

*Figure 11.24* A slight depression at the tip of the nose after cryoprobe treatment of a spider naevus – mainly epidermal atrophy. Treatment by sharp-tip hyfrecation with brief coagulation of the underlying feeder vessel often gives a better cosmetic outcome in treating spider angiomas on the face.

presented evidence to suggest that short freeze times may sometimes cause "resorption" and permanent loss of follicles without surrounding scarring, whereas "tumor regimens" lead to overall dermal damage with associated follicular scarring (**Figure 11.27**).[8] The permanence of this loss suggests that the dermal papillae are irrevocably damaged by the freezing methods used in clinical practice.

## NAIL CHANGES

Cryosurgery can be used to treat digital mucus cysts (myxoid cysts) of the distal digit (see Chapter 8). These cysts often overlie the nail matrix and create nail changes through the pressure that they exert on the matrix. At the time of diagnosis it is not unusual to see an indentation in the nail plate distal to the mucus cyst. If cryosurgery is used to treat the cyst, additional damage to the nail matrix can result in transverse nail ridges or nail shedding (**Figures 11.28 and 11.29**). Although it is theoretically possible to cause nail changes from the treatment of periungual warts, this is not a common side effect of cryosurgery. A rare event is damage to the extensor tendons of the terminal phalanx after aggressive cryosurgery.

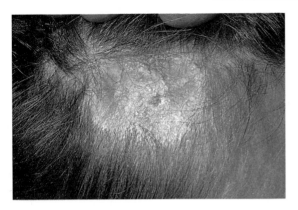

*Figure 11.27* Scarring of the scalp after treatment of a basal cell carcinoma. In general, cryosurgery is rarely a treatment of choice for scalp cancers, especially when the area of the scalp is hair bearing.

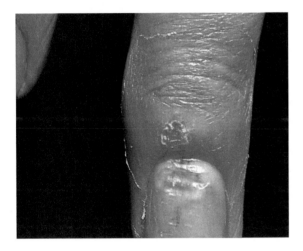

*Figure 11.28* Transverse nail ridges/furrows after cryosurgery of a digital mucous (myxoid) cyst. The cysts alone often cause ridging of the nail by their pressure on the nail matrix.

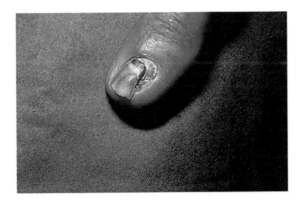

*Figure 11.29* Nail shedding after cryosurgery of a digital mucous (myxoid) cyst.cyst.

## CONCLUSION

Cryosurgery has the potential to cause immediate side effects as well as long-term complications. Good technique can prevent only some of these effects because many of the adverse effects are expected with the standard treatment process. Fortunately most side effects are temporary and long-term side effects are acceptable to patients wanting to have their skin cancers eradicated. Informed consent and good doctor–patient communication can lessen the anxiety and psychological distress that may accompany these effects. The benefits of cryosurgery are great, so expert handling of risks will see that the benefits outweigh the risks.

## REFERENCES

1. Thai KE, Fergin P, Freeman M, et al. A prospective study of the use of cryosurgery for the treatment of actinic keratoses. Int J Dermatol 2004;43:687–92.
2. Thissen MR, Nieman FH, Ideler AH, Berretty PJ, Neumann HA. Cosmetic results of cryosurgery versus surgical excision for primary uncomplicated basal cell carcinomas of the head and neck. Dermatol Surg 2000;26:759–64.
3. Jaramillo-Ayerbe F. Cryosurgery in difficult-to-treat basal cell carcinoma. Int J Dermatol 2000;39:223–9.
4. Peikert JM. Prospective trial of curettage and cryosurgery in the management of non-facial, superficial, and minimally invasive basal and squamous cell carcinoma. Int J Dermatol 2011;50:1135–8.
5. Sonnex TS, Jones RL, Weddell AG, Dawber RP. Long-term effects of cryosurgery on cutaneous sensation. Br Med J (Clin Res Ed) 1985;290:188–90.
6. Faber WR, Naafs B, Smitt JH. Sensory loss following cryosurgery of skin lesions. Br J Dermatol 1987; 117:343–7.
7. Shepherd JP, Dawber RP. Wound healing and scarring after cryosurgery. Cryobiology 1984;21:157–69.
8. Burge SM, Dawber RP. Hair follicle destruction and regeneration in guinea-pig skin after cutaneous freeze injury. Cryobiology 1990;27:153–63.

# APPENDIX A    Coding and billing pearls

The following information applies only to the US health-care system.

When cryosurgery is used for tissue destruction then coding is based on the skin destruction codes. Benign, premalignant, and malignant tissue destruction has essentially been divided into four types of CPT codes based on these diagnoses:

1. Skin tags – 11200, 11201
2. Benign other than skin tags or cutaneous vascular lesions (includes warts and seborrheic keratoses) – 17110, 17111
3. Premalignant (actinic keratoses) – 17000, 17003, 17004
4. Malignant – destruction codes based on size of lesion and location.

For destruction of skin tags, benign or premalignant lesions, size does not make a difference in coding. Location matters only for benign and malignant lesions and not for skin tags or actinic keratoses (AKs).

## SKIN TAGS
11200  Removal of skin tags by cryosurgery or any other technique, any area, up to and including 15 (billed once only)
11201  Removal for each additional 10 lesions or portion thereof (may be billed more than once)

Insurance companies in the USA will usually not pay for removal of skin tags. Sometimes documented medical reasons such as strangulation, pain, bleeding, or blocking of vision will result in reimbursement. When patients just don't like the way the skin tags look or feel, it is usually considered a cosmetic removal. In this instance, patients should be advised in advance that they will be responsible for payment and an estimate should be given. Interestingly, an office visit E/M code can be charged to insurance but the removal fee is the patient's responsibility. Documenting a medical reason is no guarantee that the insurance company will reimburse for skin tags.

## WARTS AND OTHER BENIGN LESIONS
17110  Cryosurgery (destruction by any means) of warts/benign lesions other than skin tags, up to 14 lesions (this is a single code used once only regardless if 1 or 14 lesions are treated)

17111  15 or more lesions (stand-alone code, not per lesion)

For destructions of benign lesions, there are certain specific parts of the body that are reimbursed at a higher rate including the anus, penis, vulva, vagina, and eyelid. The CPT codes, typical fees charged and average Medicare reimbursement for these are detailed in Table A.1. Don't forget to use these codes, because they do pay better than 17110 and 17111. These specific location codes are not based on the exact number of lesions and a single lesion may be reimbursed the same as many lesions.

*Table A.1* Selected Benign Skin Destructions Codes by Location

| CPT | Description | 2013 Medicare fee schedule[a] (US$) | Relative value units (RVUs) |
|-----|-------------|-------------------|-------------------|
| 46916 | Anus, cryo, simple | 238.16 | 1.91 |
| 46924 | Anus, extensive lesions | 563.76 | 2.81 |
| 54056 | Penis, cryosurgery | 145.96 | 1.29 |
| 56501 | Vulva, simple | 134.05 | 1.58 |
| 56515 | Vulva, extensive | 228.63 | 3.08 |
| 57061 | Vaginal lesion, simple | 116.70 | 1.30 |
| 57065 | Vaginal lesion, ext | 196.65 | 2.66 |
| 67850 | Lesion, eyelid | 222.17 | 1.74 |

[a]Medicare fee schedule and RVU data as of December 2013 – the Geographic Practice Cost Index (GPCI) will affect local Medicare allowable fees.

## ACTINIC KERATOSES (ICD-9 CODE 702.0)
CPT codes for cryosurgery of AKs are:

17000  Cryosurgery AK first lesion
17003  Second through 14th lesion (this code is billed for each lesion from 2 to 14 with a charge for each lesion)
17004  15 or more lesions (stand alone code, not per lesion)

Table A.2 gives for a comparison of Medicare fees and RVUs for the cryosurgery of benign and premalignant lesions.

*Table A.2* Destruction of Benign and Premalignant Lesions (Codes and Fee Schedule)

| CPT | Description | 2013 Medicare fee schedule[a] (US$) | Relative value units (RVUs) |
|---|---|---|---|
| 17110 | Benign, other than skin tags or cut vascular lesions ≤14 milia, seborrheic keratoses, warts | 114.32 | 0.70 |
| 17111 | Benign, other than skin tags or cutaneous vascular lesions ≥15 | 135.41 | 0.97 |
| 17000 | Premalignant, 1 | 83.36 | 0.65 |
| 17003 | Premalignant, 2–14, *each* | 6.80 | 0.07 |
| 17004 | Premalignant, ≥15 | 172.84 | 1.85 |

[a]Medicare Fee Schedule and RVU data as of December 2013 – the Geographic Practice Cost Index (GPCI) will affect local Medicare allowable fees.

## MALIGNANT

Destruction (including cryosurgery) codes based on size and location. In this case, the size of the lesion is the longest diameter of the lesion before treatment without the addition of a border or margin. Note that margins can be added only for surgical excision and not destruction.

17260   Trunk, arms, or legs, ≤0.5
17261   Diameter 0.6–1.0 cm
17262   Diameter 1.1–2.0 cm
17263   Diameter 2.1–3.0 cm
17270   Scalp, neck, hands, feet, or genitalia, ≤0.5 cm
17271   Diameter 0.6–1.0 cm
17272   Diameter 1.1–2.0 cm
17273   Diameter 2.1–3.0 cm
17280   Face, nose, lips, eyelids, mucous membranes, or ears, ≤0.5 cm
17281   Diameter 0.6–1.0 cm
17282   Diameter 1.1–2.0 cm
17283   Diameter 2.1–3.0 cm

It is essential to always measure the size of all malignant lesions before treatment and record this in the EMR or chart. When size is estimated rather than measured, money is often lost, eg an "eyeball estimate" of 1.0 cm will pay less than an actual measurement of 1.1 cm when the true length is 1.1 cm.

## FURTHER READING

Centers for Medicare and Medicaid. Available at: www.cms. gov/apps/physician-fee-schedule/overview.aspx (accessed March 25, 2014).

Ingenix. National Fee Analyzer. Eden Prairie, MN: Ingenix, 2010.

MAG Mutual HealthCare Solutions. Physicians' Fee & Coding Guide. Atlanta, GA: MAG Mutual HealthCare Solutions, Inc., 2010. Available at: http://coderscentral.com (accessed March 25, 2014).

Wasserman Medical Publishers. Medical coding books and software including Physician's Fee Reference. West Alice, WI: Wasserman Medical Publishers, 2010.

# APPENDIX B    Methods of learning

Our book is designed to provide in-depth knowledge of cryosurgery and step-by-step guidance in all the essential skills needed to perform a wide range of cryosurgery. Additional learning can occur while working alongside someone who is experienced in cryosurgery. However, when this is not possible, there are many workshops around the world to help learn these essential skills: determining lesions that are appropriate for cryosurgery, choosing the optimal cryosurgical instrument or tips, counseling the patient, and performing the cryosurgery. The American Academy of Family Physicians (AAFP) offers hands-on cryosurgery and electrosurgery workshops every summer and fall (see details below). The British Society for Dermatological Surgery runs an annual workshop which includes teaching of cryosurgical method. Many manufacturers of cryosurgical equipment have websites with written information and videos on how to use their equipment. Brymill cryoguns, cryoprobe, Histofreezer and other instruments come with charts of recommended freeze times for their units.

It can be very helpful to practice cryosurgical techniques on agar plates, bananas, or raw meat (chicken or beef). A clear agar plate reveals the depth and breadth of freeze when viewed from the side as the surface is frozen (Figure B.1). It helps to gain an understanding of the relationship between lateral spread and depth of freeze. Spraying evaporating liquids into a cone can take some practice to get a feel for the force and volume of spray, so it is helpful to practice it on a model before performing this on a live patient.

One ingenious model that we highly endorse is the banana which has a skin that turns brown when exposed to cold temperatures. It is easily available and can be eaten after practice. This model can be used to practice spot freezes, pulsed freezes, spiral or spray paint techniques. The following figures demonstrate the types of hands on practice one can perform with the banana model:

Figure B.2 demonstrates the breadth of spray with different tip apertures (a–d) compared with the bent tip extension and one small cryoprobe. Figure B.3 shows how one can practice using a cryospray with various geometric shapes and sizes to improve accuracy.

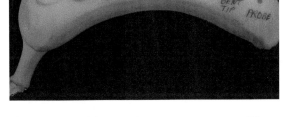

*Figure B.2* Practicing on a banana to get a sense of freeze diameters. (Courtesy of Daniel Stulberg, MD.)

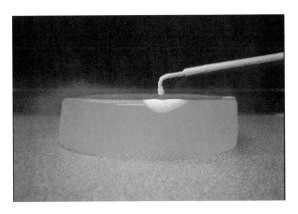

*Figure B.1* Practicing depth of freeze with an agar plate. (Courtesy of Daniel Stulberg, MD.)

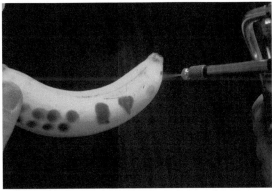

*Figure B.3* Freezing multiple lesions and shapes to improve accuracy and technique. (Courtesy of Daniel Stulberg, MD.)

Figure B.4 demonstrates the use of marked areas on the banana and the bent tip extension to stay within the marked borders. Figure B.5 demonstrates how the lateral spread of the spray may go outside the border when a small lesion is frozen if a careful intermittent spray is not utilized. Figure B.6 demonstrates the practice of using a cryoprobe with liquid nitrogen. The plastic ventilation tube should not touch the patient and should be directed away from the skin.

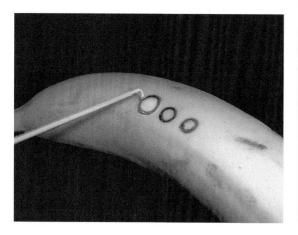

*Figure B.4* Circles marked on the banana can help learning control of the cryospray. The bent tip extension allows for great accuracy to stay within the marked borders. (Courtesy of Richard Usatine, MD.)

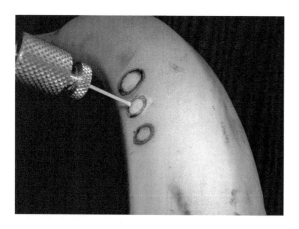

*Figure B.5* Lateral spread of the spray may go outside the intended border when a small lesion is frozen if a careful intermittent spray is not utilized. (Courtesy of Richard Usatine, MD.)

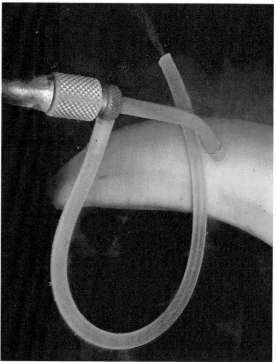

*Figure B.6* Practicing the use of a cryoprobe with liquid nitrogen and the banana model. The plastic ventilation tube should not touch the patient and should be directed away from the skin. (Courtesy of Richard Usatine, MD.)

### RESOURCES TO LEARN CRYOSURGERY

- AAFP course "Skin problems and diseases" which includes one combined cryosurgery and electrosurgery workshop: www.aafp.org/cme
- AAFP annual scientific assembly has multiple combined cryosurgery and electrosurgery workshops every fall: www.aafp.org/events/assembly.html
- The British Society for Dermatological Surgery annual workshop in April or May: www.bsds.org.uk
- Brymill videos: www.brymill.com/brymill-videos.html

# APPENDIX C    Dermoscopy

Dermoscopy allows the clinician to visualize structures below the level of the stratum corneum. These structures are not routinely discernible without dermoscopy. The presence or absence of specific dermoscopic structures, their location, and their distribution can assist the clinician in making a diagnosis or at least in narrowing the differential diagnosis.

The major goal of dermoscopy is to differentiate benign from malignant lesions on the skin so that one is less likely to miss a skin cancer (higher sensitivity) and less likely to perform unnecessary biopsies (higher specificity). Together, this will increase your diagnostic accuracy.

Dermatoscopes are currently manufactured by 3Gen, Welch Allyn, and Canfield and Heine. A number of dermatoscopes work well while attached to smart phones and cameras for easy image capture and full screen images that can be shown to the patients. There are a number of methods to use dermoscopic structures to aid in diagnosis. We prefer the two-step dermoscopy algorithm described in Figure C.1.

Dermoscopy allows the clinician to recognize suspicious features of melanomas, basal cell carcinomas, and squamous cell carcinomas. Also, benign patterns of normal nevi can be seen through the dermoscope. Many benign tumors have specific features that help to confirm the clinical impression that a lesion is a dermatofibroma, seborrheic keratosis, or angioma. This can be of great help when deciding whether to offer cryosurgery to a patient without a biopsy-proven diagnosis. Also, the visualization of a suspicious feature will help the clinician choose a biopsy over cryosurgery to avoid inadvertent treatment of a malignant lesion as a benign entity.

## RESOURCES TO LEARN DERMOSCOPY

Dermoscopy. Website from Italy that includes a free dermoscopy tutorial: www.dermoscopy.org.

International Dermoscopy Society: www.dermoscopy-ids.org.

Johr R, Stolz W. Dermoscopy: An illustrated self-assessment guide. New York: McGraw-Hill, 2010; with an interactive app: see www.usatinemedia.com.

Marghoob A, Braun R, Kopf A. Interactive CD-ROM of Dermoscopy. London: Informa Healthcare, 2007.

Marghoob AA, Malvehy J, Braun R, eds. Atlas of Dermoscopy. 2nd edn. London: Informa Healthcare, 2012.

Marghoob A, Usatine R. Dermoscopy. In: Usatine R, Pfenninger J, Stulberg D, Small R (eds), Dermatologic and Cosmetic Procedures in Office Practice. Philadelphia, PA: Elsevier, 2012.

Marghoob AA, Usatine RP, Jaimes N. Dermoscopy. In: Usatine R, Smith M, Mayeaux EJ, Chumley H. Color Atlas of Family Medicine, 2nd edn. New York: McGraw-Hill, 2013.

Marghoob AA, Usatine RP, Jaimes N. Free dermoscopy app – Dermoscopy: Two Step Algorithm. Available on iTunes and www.usatinemedia.com. Released in 2014.

Marghoob AA, Usatine RP, Jaimes N. Dermoscopy for the family physician. Am Fam Physician. 2013 Oct 1;88:441–50.

Malvehy J, Puig S, Braun, RP, Marghoob, AA, Kopf AW. Handbook of Dermoscopy. London: Taylor & Francis, 2006.

## COURSES

- American Dermoscopy Meeting is held yearly in the summer in a national park: www.americandermoscopy.com.
- Memorial Sloan–Kettering Cancer Center holds a yearly dermoscopy workshop each fall in New York City: www.mskcc.org/events.
- American Academy of Family Physicians (AAFP) yearly fall scientific assembly offers dermoscopy workshops: www.aafp.org/events/assembly.html.
- AAFP sponsors a course on "Skin Problems and Diseases" which includes a dermoscopy workshop: www.aafp.org/cme.
- American Academy of Dermatology has many lectures and workshops at its national meetings: www.aad.org.

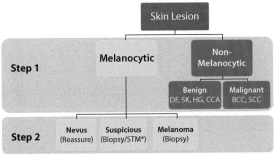

*STM: Short-term monitoring. Never monitor palpable lesions.

*Figure C.1* Two-step algorithm for dermoscopy. BCC, basal cell carcinoma; CCA, clear-cell acanthoma; DF, dermatofibroma; HG, hemangioma; SCC, squamous cell carcinoma; SK, seborrheic keratosis; STM, short-term monitoring. Never monitor palpable lesions. (By courtesy of Ashfaq A Marghoob MD and Natalia Jaimes MD.)

# Index

Page numbers in *italics* refer to figures outside of the range of the corresponding text.